Caregiver Activity Lesson Plans
Activities from the National Association of Activity Professionals - Volume 4
Activities from Wisconsin

This edition of the *Caregiver Activity Lesson Plans* features some of the favorite activities of leading Activity Professionals from around the United States. Activity Professionals are the quality of life experts that focus on the social side of long-term care and design individual programs for every resident, client or participant they work with. We have adapted those activities to make a booklet of one to one activities that can be used by any caregiver in any setting.

About Colleen Keegan

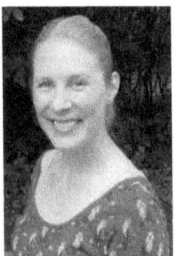

Colleen Keegan AP-BC, CDP has worked in the activity and senior care field for 12 years in various settings including adult day centers, assisted living communities and skilled nursing facilities. Colleen received her Bachelor of Fine Arts degree from the University of Wisconsin-Eau Claire, is a board certified activity professional through NAAPCC and is CDP certified through NCCDP.

About R.O.S. Therapy Systems

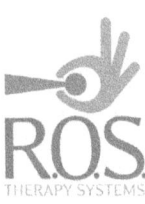

R.O.S. Therapy Systems began as a backyard project to help one family with their quality of life during a 25-year fight with Parkinson's and dementia. The company has grown into a trusted partner of quality of life tools and education for Family Caregivers, Home Care Agencies, Adult Day Centers, Assisted Living Facilities and Skilled Nursing Facilities.

ISBN

Disclaimer

This book is for informational and entertainment purposes only. All activities should be conducted under the supervision of a qualified professional, such as a Home Care Certified individual. At no time should a senior or other acting participant be left alone when conducting the activities listed in this book.

Published by
R.O.S. Therapy Systems, L.L.C.
Greensboro, NC
888-352-9788
www.ROSTherapySystems.com

How to use a Lesson Plan:

The Lesson Plan should be ever-changing. It is meant to be written on and to note any changes you may have made from the original plan so that the next person working with the participant can follow your modifications with the goal of recreating positive experiences.

Date: Document the date the activity is used with the participant

Program Name: Activity name

Objective: To provide meaningful, purposeful activities that will engage the participant

Materials: Suggested materials/resources to use with this program

Prerequisite Skills: Skills/abilities a person should possess for a particular program

Activity Outline: Step-by-step instructions to complete the program

Evaluation: A thorough evaluation is the most important part of the Lesson Plan. When conducting an activity with the participant, record any verbal cues, assistance, or modifications to incorporate into the activity. It is also helpful to include the participant's response to the program. Note if the participant dislikes a certain activity and won't ever be interested in engaging in this activity in the future.

Note programs that are successful at distracting or eliminating a negative behavior (diversion activities). Encourage family members and caregivers to use the evaluation section and also leave tips. Don't waste time recreating the wheel of knowledge; pass on the information so everyone presents the program in the same way with the same modifications and cueing, and achieving the same positive outcomes.

** A caregiver/leader must be present at all times when conducting the activities contained in this book.

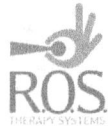 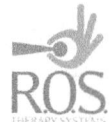

Adapting an Activity Lesson Plan

Every person has his or her own unique physical and cognitive abilities and needs. How that person responds to an activity will dictate how the leader/caregiver will continue to modify or adapt a Lesson Plan to meet individual participant's needs and abilities – now and in the future.

It is up to the leader/caregiver to determine modifications to any Activity Lesson Plan so an activity is person-centered and person-appropriate. The following activity is an example of modifying an activity:

Butterfly Craft

You know that the participant loves butterflies. You decide to use a Lesson Plan based on a butterfly craft. Depending on the participant's physical and cognitive level, you will determine what adjustments have to be made. Here are examples of four functional levels and how your butterfly activity may be modified:

- Level 1: Coffee Filter Butterfly craft: Take a coffee filter and paint it with watercolor paint. When it dries, pinch the center together and tie a pipe cleaner around the center in the shape of a butterfly body and then make two antennas.

- Level 2: Coloring pictures of butterflies

- Level 3: Looking at pictures and discussing butterflies together

- Level 4: Caregiver shows pictures of butterflies to the participant

To ensure that the participant reaps the benefits of being engaged, please adapt any and all activities to the participants functional level.

The leader should read all step-by-step directions of an Activity Outline before beginning an activity with a participant. The step-by-step directions are general guidelines for the leader/caregiver to use and potentially modify in order to help the participant successfully engage in the chosen activity.

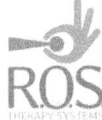 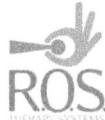

Budget and Time Saver Activities

As caregivers, our time and finances can often be strained and stretched to the limit. With that in mind, R.O.S. Therapy Systems and the National Association of Activity Professionals have designed activity lesson plans that are easy on the budget and use common household items or materials that are readily available from grocery stores or dollar stores.

Activities are not just playing Bingo; it can be anything! Here are some general activity suggestions that can help you get started and do not cost any money.

<u>Around the House Activities</u>

- Making the bed

- Folding laundry items such as napkins or towels

- Reading the newspaper

- Setting the table

- Watching a favorite television game show or program

- Having a conversation

Please remember that as a caregiver, you should be present at all times. No matter how simple YOU think an activity may be, it may be a challenge for the person you are working with and they may need assistance or some type of verbal cue. If you have designed an activity on your own or use one of the general suggestions above, please use one of the blank Lesson Plan forms at the back of this book so that all caregivers may see it. For continuity, they will need to see the notes of any verbal cues or assistance which may have been required or given for the participant to enjoy the activity.

Table of Contents

Table of Contents

Activity Lesson Plans

Indoor Gardening

Indoor Gardening Tips

- The leader must always be present when engaged in an activity.

- The leader must take all necessary and reasonable precautions to ensure the safety of the participant.

- The leader should have necessary materials ready and prepared prior to the beginning the activity.

- To ensure that the participant reaps the benefits of being engaged, please adapt any and all activities to the participants functional level.

- The leader should read all step-by-step directions of an Activity Outline before beginning an activity with a participant. The step-by-step directions are general guidelines for the leader/caregiver to use and potentially modify in order to help the participant successfully engage in the chosen activity.

- The leader must allow for the participant to be successful. The leader may have to do all prep work depending on the participant's cognitive and physical abilities. It will be up to the leader to adjust their level of involvement so that the participant does engage in these activities.

- If mistakes are made by participant - do not criticize the participant.

Program Name: Twisted Rope Flower Pots _____ **Date:** _____

Leader: _____ **Time:** _____

Objective:

- Maintain/increase motor skills
- Promote sensory, visual and tactile stimulation
- Range of motion
- Support positive thoughts of self and statements of affirmation

Materials:

- 1 package of twisted manila rope - 1/4" x 50'
- 1 empty 10 - 20 oz. coffee can
- 1 hot-glue gun
- Hot-glue gun glue sticks
- Scissors
- *Drill
- 1/8" to 1/4" drill bit for draining hole depending on size of can

*A hammer and nail can be used instead of a drill to make drainage holes in bottom of the coffee can.

Prerequisite Skills:

Every person has his or her own unique physical/cognitive abilities and needs. How a participant responds to an activity will dictate how the caregiver will modify or adapt a Lesson Plan to meet individual participant needs and abilities – now and in the future.

Program Name: Twisted Rope Flower Pots   **Date:** _____

Leader: _____   **Time:** _____

Activity Outline:

Explain to the participant that you will be making flower pots for future planting.

1. Make sure your can has multiple drainage holes for excess water. If the holes are not there, use a drill to make holes in the bottom of the can.
2. Use the hot-glue gun to glue one end of the rope to the lowest part of the side of the can.
3. Continue to use the hot-glue gun to wrap and glue, wrap and glue as you go around the can. Be sure to keep the rope pushed as close to the previously glued section as possible. This will create a beautiful rope pattern.
4. When the rope reaches the top of the can, cut off the excess rope and glue the end to the can.

Note: A hammer and nail can be used instead of a drill to make drainage holes in bottom of the coffee can.

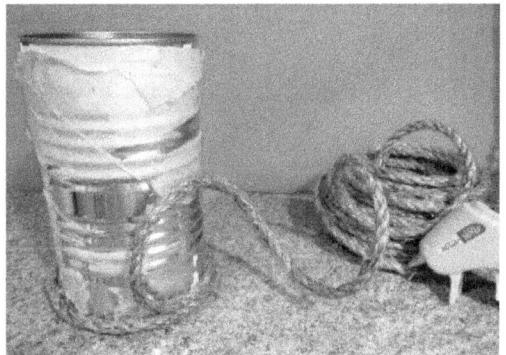

Evaluation:

Program Name: Mini Wine Cork Planters

Date: _____

Leader: _____

Time: _____

Objective:

- Maintain/increase motor skills
- Promote sensory, visual and tactile stimulation
- Range of motion
- Support positive thoughts of self and statements of affirmation

Materials:

- Tiny succulent cutting
- Wine bottle cork
- Craft knife
- Small magnet
- Common, household glue
- Dirt or potting soil - small amount

Prerequisite Skills:

Every person has his or her own unique physical/cognitive abilities and needs. How a participant responds to an activity will dictate how the caregiver will modify or adapt a Lesson Plan to meet individual participant needs and abilities – now and in the future.

Program Name: Mini Wine Cork Planters   **Date:** _____

Leader: _____   **Time:** _____

Activity Outline:

Explain to the participant that you will be making mini planters.

1. Carefully hollow out the cork with the craft knife.
2. Glue the small magnet to the back of the cork.
3. Plant your succulent cutting inside of the cork using a bit of dirt from outside or potting soil.

Note: It is important to use succulent cuttings as they are drought tolerant plants and can handle tiny amounts of soil.

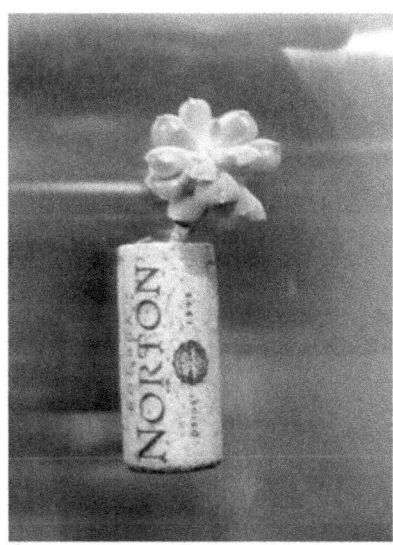

Evaluation:

Program Name: Shoe Pocket Gardens   **Date:** _____

Leader: _____   **Time:** _____

Objective:

- Maintain/increase motor skills
- Promote sensory, visual and tactile stimulation
- Range of motion
- Support positive thoughts of self and statements of affirmation

Materials:

- Hanging pocket shoe organizer
- Safety pin or push pin
- Moisture retaining soil
- Plants or seeds - lettuce, herbs & vegetables work great for this project

Prerequisite Skills:

Every person has his or her own unique physical/cognitive abilities and needs. How a participant responds to an activity will dictate how the caregiver will modify or adapt a Lesson Plan to meet individual participant needs and abilities – now and in the future.

Program Name: Shoe Pocket Gardens   **Date:** _____

Leader: _____   **Time:** _____

Activity Outline:

Explain to the participant that you will be making an indoor garden.

1. Pour water into the pockets of the shoe organizer to check the drainage. If there isn't any drainage, use the safety pin or push pin to make a few small holes in each of the pockets.
2. Add a good moisture retaining soil to each pocket. Fill to 1" below the rim so that water does not pour over the rim.
3. Add plants or seeds to each pocket.
4. Water occasionally but do not over water.

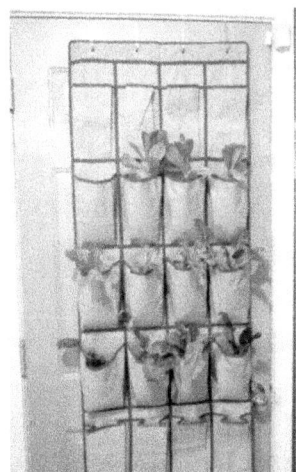 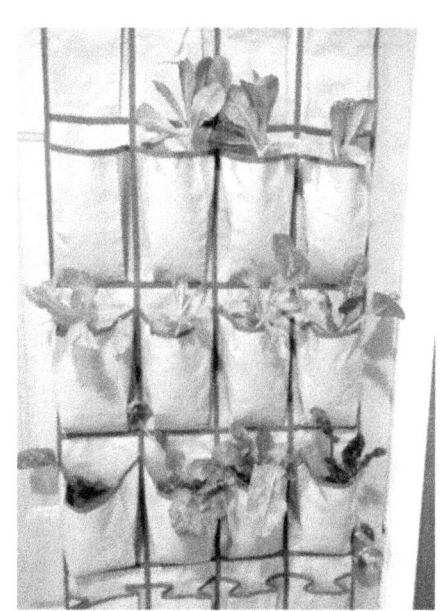

Evaluation:

Program Name: Coastal Gardens

Date: _____

Leader: _____

Time: _____

Objective:

- Maintain/increase motor skills
- Promote sensory, visual and tactile stimulation
- Range of motion
- Support positive thoughts of self and statements of affirmation

Materials:

- Small growing succulents
- A variety of large seashells, large snail shells, conch shell, clam shells, etc.
- Potting soil

Prerequisite Skills:

Every person has his or her own unique physical/cognitive abilities and needs. How a participant responds to an activity will dictate how the caregiver will modify or adapt a Lesson Plan to meet individual participant needs and abilities – now and in the future.

Program Name: Coastal Gardens   **Date:** _____

Leader: _____   **Time:** _____

Activity Outline:

Explain to the participant that you will be making seashell planters.

1. Depending on size of seashell, place a thumbful to small handful of dirt into the shell.
2. Transplant chosen succulents.

Note: These are perfect for small spaces and are very light on daily care. Keep them on the windowsill and only water them every week or so.

Note: It is important to use succulent cuttings as they are drought tolerant plants and can handle tiny amounts of soil.

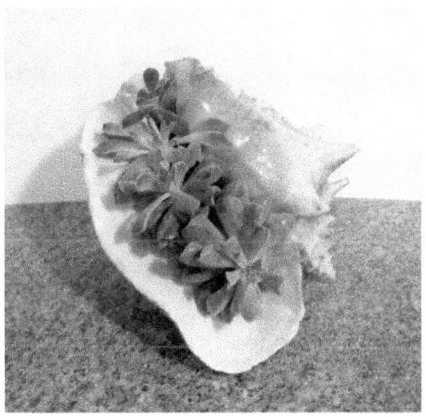

Evaluation:

Program Name: Terrarium

Date: _____

Leader: _____

Time: _____

Objective:

- Maintain/increase motor skills
- Promote sensory, visual and tactile stimulation
- Range of motion
- Support positive thoughts of self and statements of affirmation

Materials:

- Pebbles/gravel
- Activated charcoal or activated carbon (found in stores in the pet aisle - fish)
- Potting soil
- Moss
- Plants - choose your sizes wisely- you want them to fit into your container
- Clear container

Prerequisite Skills:

Every person has his or her own unique physical/cognitive abilities and needs. How a participant responds to an activity will dictate how the caregiver will modify or adapt a Lesson Plan to meet individual participant needs and abilities – now and in the future.

Program Name: Terrarium _____ **Date:** _____

Leader: _____ **Time:** _____

Activity Outline:

Explain to the participant that you will be making see through planters.

1. Add one inch of pebbles or gravel to your container.
2. Next, add a thin layer of activated charcoal.
3. Now, add the potting soil. The amount of soil will depend on the depth of the roots or bulb of the plant/flower you choose.
4. Add plant(s) and then add moss around the plants.
5. Water sparingly!

Note: If you want bright colored gravel – use fish tank gravel.

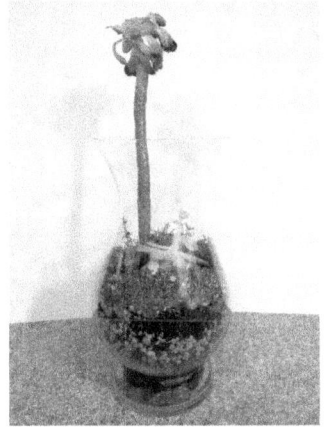 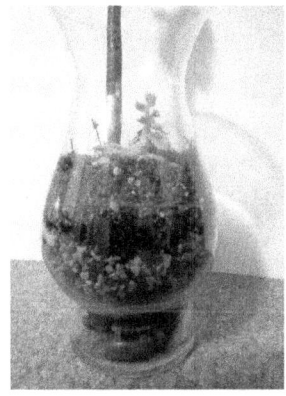

Evaluation:

Program Name: Succulent Birdhouse   **Date:** _____

Leader: _____   **Time:** _____

Objective:

- Maintain/increase motor skills
- Promote sensory, visual and tactile stimulation
- Range of motion
- Support positive thoughts of self and statements

Materials:

- Small wooden, craft birdhouse
- Acrylic paint - color of choice
- Paint brush
- Succulent cuttings
- Spanish moss
- Hot-glue gun
- Hot-glue gun glue sticks

Prerequisite Skills:

Every person has his or her own unique physical/cognitive abilities and needs. How a participant responds to an activity will dictate how the caregiver will modify or adapt a Lesson Plan to meet individual participant needs and abilities – now and in the future.

Program Name: <u>Succulent Birdhouse</u>   **Date:** _____

Leader: _____   **Time:** _____

Activity Outline:

Explain to the participant that you will be making beautiful decorative birdhouses.

1. Paint the birdhouse in your choice of colors.
2. Let the birdhouse fully dry. While drying, have a conversation about birds.
3. Use the hot-glue gun to attach the Spanish moss to the roof of the birdhouse.
4. Glue the succulent cuttings to the moss to decorate the birdhouse roof. The hot glue will not damage the succulents!
5. Plant care: Mist succulents on a weekly basis.

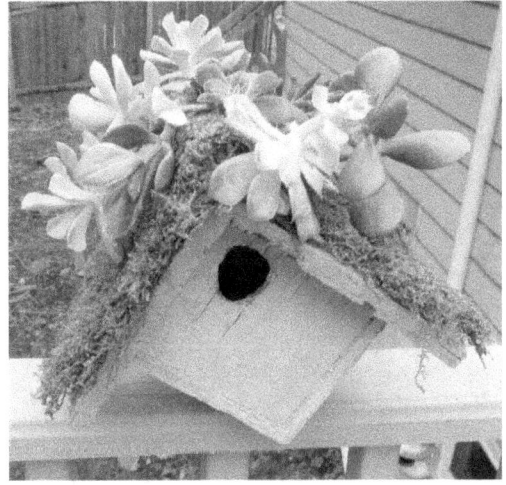

Evaluation:

Program Name: Mason Jar Herb Planters

Date: _____

Leader: _____

Time: _____

Objective:

- Maintain/increase motor skills
- Promote sensory, visual and tactile stimulation
- Range of motion
- Support positive thoughts of self and statements of affirmation

Materials:

- Herbs of your choosing
- Jars (mason, Kerr, pickle, whatever!)
- Potting soil
- Soil cover rocks
- Spoon
- Water

Prerequisite Skills:

Every person has his or her own unique physical/cognitive abilities and needs. How a participant responds to an activity will dictate how the caregiver will modify or adapt a Lesson Plan to meet individual participant needs and abilities – now and in the future.

Program Name: Mason Jar Herb Planters   **Date:** _____

Leader: _____   **Time:** _____

Activity Outline:

Explain to the participant that you will be making "see through" planters using mason jars.

1. Take the jars and fill the bottom 2-3 inches with the soil cover rocks. *This is very important when planting in jars because it allows the water to seep into the rocks and prevents mold growth.
2. Fill the jar about 2/3 of the way full with potting soil. A moisture control soil is your best choice.
3. Remove your herb from the container and spread the roots apart.
4. Place your herb inside of the jar and on top of the potting soil.
5. Add more potting soil around the herb. Use a spoon if necessary.
6. Pack the soil.
7. Water your plant - when you water the herb, the soil will settle.

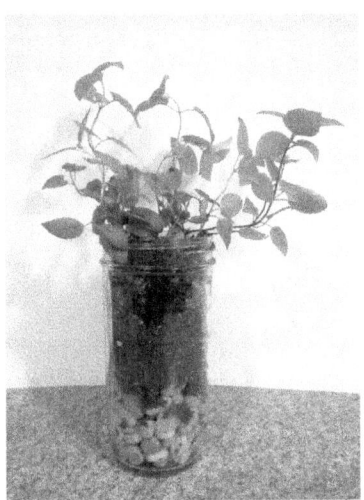
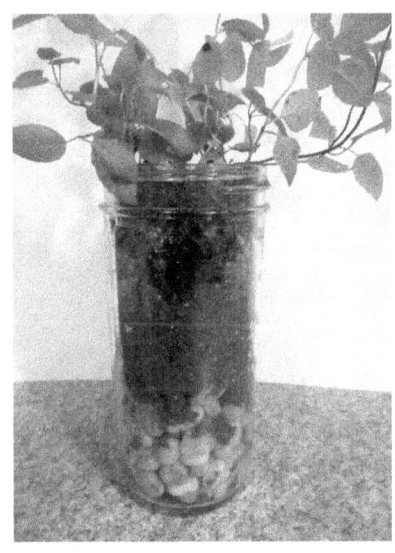

Evaluation:

Program Name: Vintage Toolbox Garden   **Date:** _____

Leader: _____   **Time:** _____

Objective:

- Maintain/increase motor skills
- Promote sensory, visual and tactile stimulation
- Range of motion
- Support positive thoughts of self and statements of affirmation

Materials:

- Vintage toolbox (or plant box)
- *Drill
- *1/4" drill bit
- Liner - pebbles, gravel, stones or clay brick pieces
- Potting soil- be sure to use a loose, light, quick-drying potting soil
- Selection of succulents

* A hammer and nail can be used instead of drill to make drainage holes in bottom of the toolbox

Prerequisite Skills:

Every person has his or her own unique physical/cognitive abilities and needs. How a participant responds to an activity will dictate how the caregiver will modify or adapt a Lesson Plan to meet individual participant needs and abilities – now and in the future.

Program Name: Vintage Toolbox Garden   **Date:** _____

Leader: _____   **Time:** _____

Activity Outline:

Explain to the participant that you will be making a vintage toolbox garden.

1. Make sure your box has multiple drainage holes for excess water. If the box does not have any drainage holes, use a drill to make holes in the bottom of toolbox.
2. Select a liner to fill the bottom of your box and lay it down.
3. Add soil and be sure to not pack the soil in too tight. Leave about 3″ at the top for your succulents.
4. Pot your succulents into your box, leaving space in between the plants for growth.
5. Once you've finished potting your plants, water lightly.

Note: A hammer and nail can be used instead of drill to make drainage holes in bottom of tool box.

Evaluation:

Program Name: Tin Can Planters   **Date:** _____

Leader: _____   **Time:** _____

Objective:

- Maintain/increase motor skills
- Promote sensory, visual and tactile stimulation
- Range of motion
- Support positive thoughts of self and statements of affirmation

Materials:

- Tin cans (washed and dried very well)
- Hammer
- Nail
- Spray paint (outdoor water and rust resistant)
- Succulents or other small plants
- Soil
- Rocks
- Flowers

Prerequisite Skills:

Every person has his or her own unique physical/cognitive abilities and needs. How a participant responds to an activity will dictate how the caregiver will modify or adapt a Lesson Plan to meet individual participant needs and abilities – now and in the future.

Program Name: Tin Can Planters   **Date:** _____

Leader: _____   **Time:** _____

Activity Outline:

Explain to the participant that you will be making tin can planters.

1. Prep the can(s) - be sure the can is free of any metal shards left over from opening it. Wash and dry the can. Remove any labels using hot water and dish soap.
2. Use the hammer and nail to place drainage holes in the bottom of each can.
3. Using spray paint, spray the cans. Spray the outside and bottom of the can first and let dry. (approximately 20-30 minutes)
4. Place rocks at the bottom for drainage.
5. Add soil.
6. Plant your flowers!

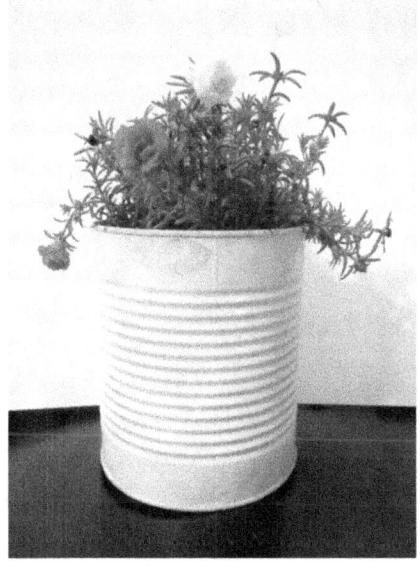 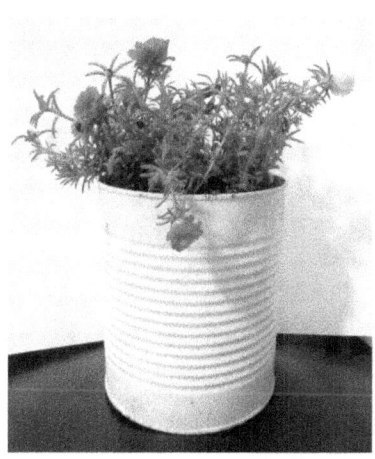

Evaluation:

Activity Lesson Plans

Indoor / Outdoor Natural Art

Indoor / Outdoor Natural Art Tips

- The leader must always be present when engaged in an activity.

- The leader must take all necessary and reasonable precautions to ensure the safety of the participant.

- The leader should have necessary materials ready and prepared prior to beginning the activity.

- To ensure that the participant reaps the benefits of being engaged, please adapt any and all activities to the participant's functional level.

- The leader should read all step-by-step directions of an Activity Outline before beginning an activity with a participant. The step-by-step directions are general guidelines for the leader/caregiver to use and potentially modify in order to help the participant successfully engage in the chosen activity.

- The leader must allow for the participant to be successful. The leader may have to do all prep work depending on the participant's cognitive and physical abilities. It will be up to the leader to adjust their level of involvement so that the participant does engage in these activities.

- If mistakes are made by participant - do not criticize the participant.

Program Name: Leaf Relief Art _____ **Date:** _____

Leader: _____ **Time:** _____

Objective:

- Maintain/increase motor skills
- Tactile and visual stimulation
- Range of motion

Materials:

- 1 box of gelatin
- Toothpick
- Cookie sheet
- Printmaking brayer (sold in most craft stores)
- Printing ink
- Variety of leaves
- Paper - slightly larger than the cookie sheet

Prerequisite Skills:

Every person has his or her own unique physical/cognitive abilities and needs. How a participant responds to an activity will dictate how the caregiver will modify or adapt a Lesson Plan to meet individual participant needs and abilities – now and in the future.

Program Name: Leaf Relief Art _____   **Date:** _____

Leader: _____   **Time:** _____

Activity Outline:

Activity Preparation

1. The night before the project, the leader will need to prepare the sheets of gelatin. Follow the measurements on the box and be sure to whisk apart any clumps of the gelatin. If there are any clumps you cannot break apart, remove them with a spoon.
2. Pour the gelatin mixture into a cookie sheet, filling it about 1".
3. Leave the sheet uncovered over night. If you see any bubbles in the gelatin on the cookie sheet, pop them with a toothpick.

Explain to the participant that you will be making leaf art.

1st Print -

1. Using a brayer and printing ink, cover the surface of the gelatin in ink. Roll the brayer back and forth until the ink is spread evenly across the surface.
2. Arrange your leaves onto the cookie sheet - veiny side down.
3. Lay one piece of paper on top of the cookie sheet and rub the back of the paper with the brayer - be sure to apply pressure to each section of your paper for an even print.
4. Pull the paper off of the cookie sheet and you have your first print!

2nd Print -

1. Carefully remove all of the leaves from the tray - it is easiest to remove the leaves by pulling at the end of their stems. You do not want to puncture the gelatin, as the hole will then fill with ink and print a black hole onto your final print.
2. Place a new sheet of paper over the empty cookie sheet and rub.
3. Pull the second print from the cookie sheet and you will have a positive image of the first print!

Once both prints have been pulled, re-ink the cookie sheet and repeat steps 2 through 7 for additional prints.

Evaluation:

Program Name: Leaf and Flower Pounding Bookmarks   **Date:** _____

Leader: _____   **Time:** _____

Objective:

- Maintain/increase motor skills
- Tactile and visual stimulation
- Range of motion

Materials:

- Light colored cardstock or watercolor paper
- Variety of fresh picked flowers and leaves (You will want to use flowers with a high amount of pigment. Examples of this are pansies, violets, peonies petals, rose petals, phlox, impatiens, geraniums, St. Johns wort and forget-me-nots).
- Hard surface for hammering - chopping board, clipboard or a strong table that will not dent when gently hit with a hammer
- Lightweight hammer or rubber mallet
- Tape
- Paper towel
- Butter knife or tweezers

Prerequisite Skills:

Every person has his or her own unique physical/cognitive abilities and needs. How a participant responds to an activity will dictate how the caregiver will modify or adapt a Lesson Plan to meet individual participant needs and abilities – now and in the future.

Program Name: Leaf and Flower Pounding Bookmarks   **Date:** _____

Leader: _____   **Time:** _____

Activity Outline:

Explain to the participant that you will be making leaf and flower bookmarks.

1. Gather the flowers and leaves that you will be using.
2. Tape the cardstock to the hard surface. This will prevent the paper from moving during the transfer.
3. Choose an area of the cardstock to begin working and arrange some of the flowers and leaves face down.
4. Place a paper towel over the flowers and leaves and tape the paper towel into place so it does not move during the transfer.
5. Carefully pound the flowers and leaves with a hammer or rubber mallet. As you gently pound, the pigment from the flowers and leaves will soak into the paper. The longer you pound, the more the pigment will be transferred to the paper.
6. When you are finished pounding, peel the paper towel from the paper.
7. Using a butter knife or a tweezers, remove the flowers and leaves from the paper.
8. Let the print dry for 10 minutes.

Note: There are many different uses for flower pounded prints beyond bookmarks - greeting cards, art prints, wrapping paper, and this process can also be used on fabric!

Evaluation:

Program Name: Seed Bombs   **Date:** _____

Leader: _____   **Time:** _____

Objective:

- Maintain/increase motor skills
- Tactile and visual stimulation
- Range of motion

Materials:

- Wildflower seeds (4 - 5 packets)
- Air dry clay
- Garden soil (or dirt from your yard)
- Water
- Parchment paper
- Cookie sheet
- Large mixing bowl

Prerequisite Skills:

Every person has his or her own unique physical/cognitive abilities and needs. How a participant responds to an activity will dictate how the caregiver will modify or adapt a Lesson Plan to meet individual participant needs and abilities – now and in the future.

Program Name: Seed Bombs   **Date:** _____

Leader: _____   **Time:** _____

Activity Outline:

Explain to the participant that you will be making seed bombs to plant for beautiful flower beds.

1. Mix 5 parts clay to 2 parts dirt in a large mixing bowl.
2. Pour in the wildflower seeds and a tiny amount of water and start mixing together with your hands. You can add more water in small amounts as you go along if the mixture is too dry.
3. Continue to mix the dirt mixture with your hands and break up any clumps of clay or dirt as you mix. If the mixture is too dry, add a little more water, if it is too wet, add more soil. You want the consistency to be similar to cookie dough.
4. Once the mixture resembles the consistency of cookie dough, take small handfuls of the mixture and roll them into balls.
5. Set the balls aside on a cookie sheet lined with parchment paper.
6. Let dry for 1-2 days. The amount of drying time will depend on the humidity level in your area.
7. Once the seed balls are dry, you can package them up as gifts or toss a few on the ground and wait for them to grow!

Note: This activity gets a bit messy - recommendation - do activity outside or near a sink.
Note: The measurements above are an estimation and the amount of water may vary. It is up to the leader to determine the final amounts based on how moist your soil is.

Evaluation:

Program Name: Sun Prints   **Date:** _____

Leader: _____   **Time:** _____

Objective:

- Maintain/increase motor skills
- Tactile and visual stimulation
- Range of motion

Materials:

- White, 100% cotton fabric
- Acrylic paint (choose 3-4 colors, darker hues will work best)
- Freshly picked flowers and leaves
- Plastic sheet or a garbage bag
- 1 piece of cardboard that is larger than your cloth
- Small, disposable cups (the same number as the amount of paint colors you will be using)
- Paintbrush
- Scissors
- Water

Prerequisite Skills:

Every person has his or her own unique physical/cognitive abilities and needs. How a participant responds to an activity will dictate how the caregiver will modify or adapt a Lesson Plan to meet individual participant needs and abilities – now and in the future.

Program Name: Sun Prints   **Date:** _____

Leader: _____   **Time:** _____

Activity Outline:

Explain to the participant that you will be making sun prints.

1. Gather a variety of fresh flower and leaves. Look for different shapes and sizes, but remember that flowers and leaves that lie flat will be the easiest to work with.
2. Cover your piece of cardboard with the plastic sheeting (or garbage bag) - this will be your workspace!
3. Dampen your cotton cloth with water and then wring it out until the cloth no longer drips. Lay the fabric flat on top of your workspace.
4. Take the paints you have chosen and place a few drops of each color in each of the small, disposable cups. Add water to the cups to dilute the paint - dilute one part paint to one part water.
5. Being sure that the fabric is still wet, paint the different colors onto the fabric until the fabric is completely covered. Be creative! Use different brushstrokes and patterns when applying the paint.
6. While the paint is still wet, arrange the flowers and leaves onto the fabric. Be sure to lay the flowers and leaves flat and press the edges down as much as possible. This will give you a clear, defined edge after they have been removed.
7. Place your workspace in the sunshine for one hour.
8. After the paint is dry, remove the flowers and leaves from the top of the fabric. The fabric will contain the beautiful silhouettes of the flowers and leaves that you had arranged on your fabric!

Note: This activity will only be successful on sunny days!

Evaluation:

Program Name: <u>Clay Leaf Bowls</u>   **Date:** _____

Leader: _____   **Time:** _____

Objective:

- Maintain/increase motor skills
- Tactile and visual stimulation
- Range of motion

Materials:

- Air-dry clay
- Freshly picked leaves
- Clay rolling mat
- Acrylic clay roller or rolling pin
- Clay scissors
- Aluminum foil
- Tweezers

Prerequisite Skills:

Every person has his or her own unique physical/cognitive abilities and needs. How a participant responds to an activity will dictate how the caregiver will modify or adapt a Lesson Plan to meet individual participant needs and abilities – now and in the future.

Program Name: Clay Leaf Bowls _____   **Date:** _____

Leader: _____   **Time:** _____

Activity Outline:

Explain to the participant that you will be making pottery.

1. Roll out the air-dry clay to approximately ¼" thickness on the clay mat.
2. Place one leaf, vein side down, on the surface of the clay.
3. Use the clay roller to roll directly over the leaf. This will push the leaf into the surface of the clay and thin the clay out.
4. Lift the clay off the mat, leaving the leaf in place, and trim the excess clay with scissors. At this time, you can cut a general shape around the leaf - you will be able to go back later and do detailed cutting.
5. Use the aluminum foil to create an oval shaped ring. Gently arrange the leaf covered clay inside - make sure the bottom of the clay is resting on a flat surface - this will ensure that the bowl will sit upright once it is dry.
6. Use the tweezers to gently remove the leaf from the clay.
7. Let the clay dry overnight.
8. Remove the clay from the aluminum foil ring and turn the bowl over so that the bottom is able to dry.
9. Optional: Use acrylic, watercolor or tempera paint to add color to your bowl.

Evaluation:

Program Name: Seashell Wall Hanging   **Date:** _____

Leader: _____   **Time:** _____

Objective:

- Maintain/increase motor skills
- Tactile and visual stimulation
- Range of motion

Materials:

- An assortment of seashells
- A creative base for your art - some examples are a sheet of sandpaper, a small shadowbox, a small wood pallet or colored cardstock.
- Mini hot-glue gun
- Glue sticks for mini hot-glue gun

Prerequisite Skills:

Every person has his or her own unique physical/cognitive abilities and needs. How a participant responds to an activity will dictate how the caregiver will modify or adapt a Lesson Plan to meet individual participant needs and abilities – now and in the future.

Program Name: Seashell Wall Hanging   **Date:** _____

Leader: _____   **Time:** _____

Activity Outline:

Explain to the participant that you will be making ocean themed art.

1. Choose the shape you would like to create with your seashells.
2. Arrange the seashells into this shape by laying them on top of your chosen base.
3. Pick the shells up one at a time and use the hot-glue gun to add a small amount of glue to the back of the shell before placing it back on the base.
4. Repeat Step 3 until every shell has been glued to the base.
5. Let dry for 20 minutes.
6. Hang for display!

Evaluation:

Program Name: Will-Not-Wilt Cactus   **Date:** _____

Leader: _____   **Time:** _____

Objective:

- Maintain/increase motor skills
- Tactile and visual stimulation
- Range of motion

Materials:

- River stones
- Small stones
- Various shades of green acrylic paint
- Paint brush
- White permanent markers
- Pot of soil

Prerequisite Skills:

Every person has his or her own unique physical/cognitive abilities and needs. How a participant responds to an activity will dictate how the caregiver will modify or adapt a Lesson Plan to meet individual participant needs and abilities – now and in the future.

Program Name: Will-Not-Wilt Cactus _____ **Date:** _____

Leader: _____ **Time:** _____

Activity Outline:

Explain to the participant that you will be making desert themed art.

1. Paint the river stones different shades of green.
2. Let the paint dry.
3. Using the white markers, draw cactus barbs onto the river stones.
4. Place the small rocks on top of the pot of soil, forming a rock base.
5. Add the river rocks vertically into the container to form the shape of a cactus.

Evaluation:

Program Name: Heart Shaped Topiary   **Date:** _____

Leader: _____   **Time:** _____

Objective:

- Maintain/increase motor skills
- Tactile and visual stimulation
- Range of motion

Materials:

- Ivy with roots
- Copper water line or thick wire
- Wire cutters
- Pot
- Rocks
- Sand
- Potting Soil
- Trowel
- Water

Prerequisite Skills:

Every person has his or her own unique physical/cognitive abilities and needs. How a participant responds to an activity will dictate how the caregiver will modify or adapt a Lesson Plan to meet individual participant needs and abilities – now and in the future.

Program Name: Heart Shaped Topiary   **Date**: _____

Leader: _____   **Time**: _____

Activity Outline:

Explain to the participant that you will be making a beautiful topiary.

1. Bend the copper piping into a heart shape. You can use the rim of the pot to bend perfect curves.
2. Use the wire cutters to snip off any excess copper frame, but be sure that you have allowed for an extra few inches to be buried under the soil.
3. Place some rocks in the bottom of the pot and insert the copper heart into the pot and down into the rocks as far as possible.
4. Using a trowel, add sand on top of the rocks and around the copper frame to add stability.
5. Add a layer of soil on top of the sand, but do not completely fill the pot.
6. Add the ivy clippings to the center of the pot and at the middle of the heart frame.
7. Cover the roots of the ivy clippings with potting soil. Fill the pot with soil until you reach just below the rim.
8. Press down on the soil to compact it against the roots. Add more soil if needed.
9. Wrap and train the ivy clippings around the copper frame. *If some of the ivy strands will not stay around the copper frame, you can use string, a twisty tie or floral wire to secure them.
10. Topiary care - Water your ivy topiary and set in a sunny spot. As the ivy continues to grow and sends out more shoots, train the new shoots around the copper frame or pinch off any shoots you wish to remove.

Evaluation:

Program Name: Botanical Ice Lantern   **Date:** _____

Leader: _____   **Time:** _____

Objective:

- Maintain/increase motor skills
- Tactile and visual stimulation
- Range of motion

Materials:

- Two containers of different sizes - such as an 18 ounce and 6 ounce jar or different sized tin cans - be sure there is at least ½" space on either side and at the bottom of the smaller container.
- Decorative filler such as:
    - orange slices
    - cranberries
    - cedar branches
    - pine needles
    - juniper berries
- Electrical tape
- Small rocks
- Water
- Battery-operated tealight candle

Prerequisite Skills:

Every person has his or her own unique physical/cognitive abilities and needs. How a participant responds to an activity will dictate how the caregiver will modify or adapt a Lesson Plan to meet individual participant needs and abilities – now and in the future.

Program Name: Botanical Ice Lantern   **Date:** _____

Leader: _____   **Time:** _____

Activity Outline:

Explain to the participant that you will be making an ice lantern.

1. Put a small amount of water into the larger container (about ½ cup).
2. Place the smaller container inside of the larger container. The smaller container should be floating inside of the larger container.
3. Add a few rocks into the smaller container to hold it down and to match the level of the larger container.
4. Add tape onto four sides of the smaller container to help hold the smaller container in the center of the larger container.
5. Place your greenery and decorative items down into the water in-between the two containers. *Berries will float to the top, so either keep them attached in sprigs or place them first into the side of the container.
6. Add more water between the containers until the water is about ½" below the top of the can. *Remember that the water will expand as it freezes so do not fill the container too full or it will overflow as it turns into ice.
7. If the temperature is below freezing where you live, simply place the containers outside overnight. If not, place them in your freezer overnight.
8. To remove the lanterns from their containers, run slightly warm water over the outside of the largest container as well as inside the smaller container to loosen the ice.
9. Once the outside begins to melt, you will be able to slide the ice lantern right out of the container mold.
10. Place a small, battery operated, tealight candle into the lantern and enjoy the beautiful glow! These lanterns can be made in various sizes using different sized containers and look gorgeous lined in front of a home or down a driveway or walkway!

Evaluation:

Program Name: Moss Graffiti _____   **Date:** _____

Leader: _____   **Time:** _____

Objective:

- Maintain/increase motor skills
- Tactile and visual stimulation
- Range of motion

Materials:

- Moss (1 or 2 small clumps)
- 2 cups of buttermilk OR plain yogurt
- 2 cups of water
- ½ teaspoon sugar
- Blender
- Paint brush
- Corn syrup
- Large container to hold final mixture
- Object to graffiti - there are many possibilities! You can paint on concrete or rough wooden walls, on rough wooden signs, pots, dishes and sculptures.

Prerequisite Skills:

Every person has his or her own unique physical/cognitive abilities and needs. How a participant responds to an activity will dictate how the caregiver will modify or adapt a Lesson Plan to meet individual participant needs and abilities – now and in the future.

Program Name: Moss Graffiti _____ **Date:** _____

Leader: _____ **Time:** _____

Activity Outline:

Explain to the participant that you will be making graffiti art.

1. Add 2 cups of water and 2 cups of either buttermilk or plain yogurt to the blender.
2. Add 2 clumps of moss to the blender - it is ok if you have to break the clumps into smaller pieces to fit them inside of the blender. *Be sure to remove as much dirt as possible from the moss before adding it to the blender.
3. Blend until the mixture is completely smooth - similar to a paint consistency. If the mixture becomes too thin and liquefies, simply add corn syrup. You will need the moss cells intact for the graffiti to work.
4. Transfer the mixture to a container to use while painting.
5. Apply the moss paint to a textured or porous surface for the best results. *Warning: This mixture will remove paint from walls.
6. After you have completed painting, mist the moss daily for several weeks until the moss begins to grow. *If you live in a particularly dry climate, you will want to mist more often so that the moss does not dry out. Too much sun will also dry out your moss - pick a moderately sunny location for your art.

Caring for your Art - Spray water or apply more moss mixture to keep your art alive! If you decide you wish to remove the moss from your object, simply spray with lime juice.

Evaluation:

Activity Lesson Plans

Indoor / Outdoor Games

Indoor / Outdoor Game Tips

- The leader must always be present when engaged in an activity.

- The leader must take all necessary and reasonable precautions to ensure the safety of participant.

- The leader should have necessary materials ready and prepared prior to beginning the activity.

- To ensure that the participant reaps the benefits of being engaged, please adapt any and all activities to the participant's functional level.

- The leader should read all step-by-step directions of an Activity Outline before beginning an activity with a participant. The step-by-step directions are general guidelines for the leader/caregiver to use and potentially modify in order to help the participant successfully engage in the chosen activity.

- The leader must allow for the participant to be successful. The leader may have to assist depending on participant's cognitive and physical abilities. It will be up to the leader to adjust their level of involvement so that the participant does engage in these activities.

- If mistakes are made by participant, do not criticize the participant. Encourage and offer praise when necessary.

Program Name: Hula Hoop Toss   **Date:** _____

Leader: _____   **Time:** _____

Objective:

- Maintain/increase motor skills
- Promote kinesthetic, sensory, visual and tactile stimulation
- Range of motion
- Promote physical stretching and movement of muscles

Materials:

- 4 - 6 hula hoops
- 4 - 6 balloons
- Ribbon or string - cut 4' in length
- Black marker
- Multiple bean bags

Prerequisite Skills:

Every person has his or her own unique physical/cognitive abilities and needs. How a participant responds to an activity will dictate how the caregiver will modify or adapt a Lesson Plan to meet individual participant needs and abilities – now and in the future.

Program Name: Hula Hoop Toss   **Date:** _____

Leader: _____   **Time:** _____

Activity Outline:

Explain to the participant that you will be playing a ring toss game.

Game Preparation:
1. Inflate 4 - 6 balloons with helium at local store.
2. Cut 4 - 6 pieces of ribbon or string, one for each balloon, into 4 foot lengths.
3. Write different point values on each of the balloons (e.g. 10, 20, 30, 40).
4. Tie one end of the ribbon or string to the balloon and the other end of the string to the hula hoop.
5. Place the hula hoops in different configurations depending on skill level and physical ability, closer or farther away.

Playing the game:
1. Explain to participant that the object of game is to score points by tossing one bean bag at a time into the hula hoop they are aiming for.
2. Toss the bean bags in an attempt to have them land inside the hula hoop. If the bean bag lands inside the hula hoop, the player is rewarded the number of points written on the balloon.

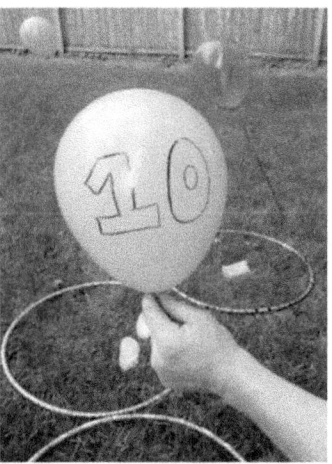 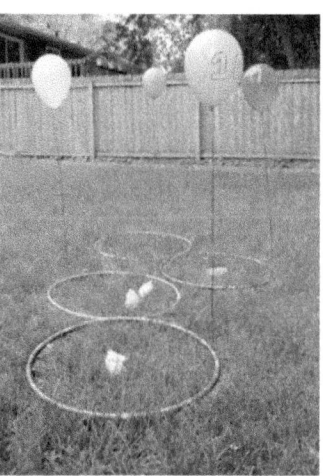

Evaluation:

Program Name: Balloon Tennis _____   **Date:** _____

Leader: _____   **Time:** _____

Objective:

- Maintain/increase motor skills
- Promote kinesthetic, sensory, visual and tactile stimulation
- Range of motion
- Promote physical stretching and movement of muscles

Materials:

- 2 paper plates
- 2 wooden painting stir sticks
- Duct tape
- 1 balloon

Prerequisite Skills:

Every person has his or her own unique physical/cognitive abilities and needs. How a participant responds to an activity will dictate how the caregiver will modify or adapt a Lesson Plan to meet individual participant needs and abilities – now and in the future.

Program Name: Balloon Tennis   **Date:** _____

Leader: _____   **Time:** _____

Activity Outline:

Explain to the participant that you will be playing indoor tennis.

Game Preparation:
1. Place the top of the paint stir stick on the back of the paper plate.
2. Using duct tape, tape the paint stir stick to the paper plate to secure them together.
3. Inflate one balloon.

Play the game:
1. Use the paper plate "rackets" to volley the balloon back and forth.

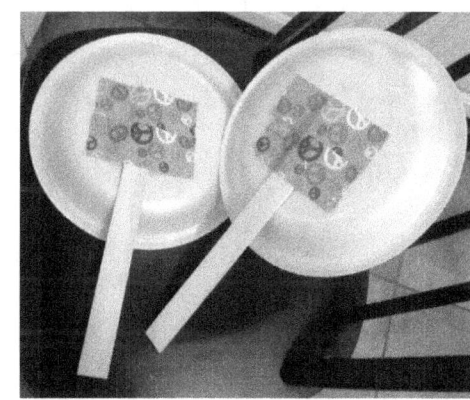

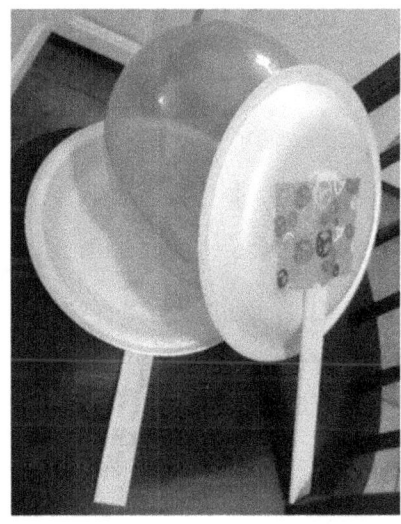

Evaluation:

Program Name: Ping Pong Darts   **Date:** _____

Leader: _____   **Time:** _____

Objective:

- Maintain/increase motor skills
- Promote kinesthetic, sensory, visual and tactile stimulation
- Range of motion
- Promote physical stretching and movement of muscles

Materials:

- Sticky backed Velcro strips
- 3 or 4 ping pong balls
- 1 sheet blue felt
- 1 sheet red felt
- 1 sheet yellow felt
- Thumbtacks
- Scissors
- Glue

Prerequisite Skills:

Every person has his or her own unique physical/cognitive abilities and needs. How a participant responds to an activity will dictate how the caregiver will modify or adapt a Lesson Plan to meet individual participant needs and abilities – now and in the future.

Program Name: Ping Pong Darts   **Date:** _____

Leader: _____   **Time:** _____

Activity Outline:

Explain to the participant that you will be playing a form of darts.

Game Preparation:
1. Cut the Velcro into several thin (about 1/2 cm) strip pieces.
2. Peel the paper backings off the hook halves of the sticky backed Velcro strips.
3. Place the hook halves of the sticky backed Velcro strips onto the ping pong balls. Make sure the Velcro covers the ball adequately so that the ball will stick well to the Velcro board when thrown.
4. Set the ping pong balls to the side.
5. Using the scissors, cut a large circle out of the sheet of yellow felt.
6. Cut a circle from the sheet of blue felt that is slightly smaller than the yellow felt circle.
7. Cut a circle out of the sheet of red felt that is smaller than the blue felt circle.
8. Apply glue to the back of the blue felt circle.
9. Press the blue felt circle onto the center of the yellow felt circle.
10. Allow the glue to dry completely.
11. Apply glue to the red felt circle.
12. Press the red felt circle onto the center of the blue felt circle.
13. Allow the glue to dry completely.
14. Hang the dry dartboard on the wall with the thumbtacks.

Play the game:
1. Explain to participant that you will be throwing the balls at the game board to make them stick.
2. To make it challenging, keep track of the points! Players who hit the red center get 10 points. The blue circle is worth 5 points and the outside yellow circle is worth 3 points.

Evaluation:

Program Name: Ladder Skeeball _____   **Date:** _____

Leader: _____   **Time:** _____

Objective:

- Maintain/increase motor skills
- Promote kinesthetic, sensory, visual and tactile stimulation
- Range of motion
- Promote physical stretching and movement of muscles

Materials:

- Ladder
- 5 sheets of printer paper
- Black marker
- Masking tape
- Multiple bean bags

Prerequisite Skills:

Every person has his or her own unique physical/cognitive abilities and needs. How a participant responds to an activity will dictate how the caregiver will modify or adapt a Lesson Plan to meet individual participant needs and abilities – now and in the future.

Program Name: Ladder Skeeball   **Date:** _____

Leader: _____   **Time:** _____

Activity Outline:

Explain to the participant that you will be playing a bag toss game.

Game Preparation:
1. Write different point values on each of the 5 different pieces of paper (e.g. 10, 20, 30, 40, 50).
2. Label each rung of a step in the ladder with one of the pieces of paper.
3. Create a "throwing line" with masking tape. The throwing line is the line from which each participant must stand or sit behind and toss the bean bag at the ladder.
4. Once the ladder rungs have been labeled with points and the throwing line created, you are ready to play the game.

Game Objective:
1. Explain to participant that the object of game is to score points by tossing one bean bag at a time at the ladder to hit the number they are aiming for.
2. Try to get as many points as possible by throwing bean bags between the rungs. Add the points up as you go along!

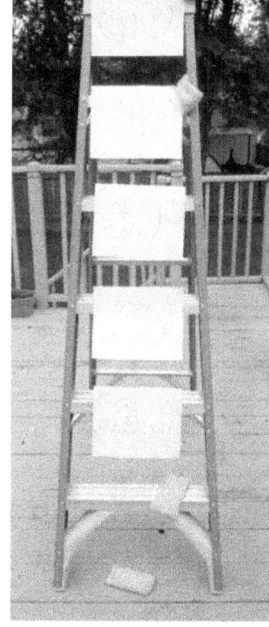

Evaluation:

Program Name: Passing Accuracy   **Date:** _____

Leader: _____   **Time:** _____

Objective:

- Maintain/increase motor skills
- Promote kinesthetic, sensory, visual and tactile stimulation
- Range of motion
- Promote physical stretching and movement of muscles

Materials:

- 1 large tarp or light colored sheet
- Duct tape - various colors
- Scissors
- Black permanent marker
- Football or other throwing ball

Prerequisite Skills:

Every person has his or her own unique physical/cognitive abilities and needs. How a participant responds to an activity will dictate how the caregiver will modify or adapt a Lesson Plan to meet individual participant needs and abilities – now and in the future.

Program Name: Passing Accuracy _____   **Date:** _____

Leader: _____   **Time:** _____

Activity Outline:

Explain to the participant that you will be playing a throwing accuracy game.

Game Preparations:
1. Lay the tarp or sheet out flat on the floor.
2. Use the scissors to cut out several different size squares in the tarp - large enough for the ball to make it through the cut outs.
3. Line the edges of the cut out squares with colorful duct tape.
4. Use the black marker to mark each square with a different point value.

Play the Game:
1. Attempt to throw the ball through the squares to earn points.
2. Make it fun by seeing who can get the most points in 10 throws.

Evaluation:

Program Name: Disc Tic Tac Toss   **Date:** _____

Leader: _____   **Time:** _____

Objective:

- Maintain/increase motor skills
- Promote kinesthetic, sensory, visual and tactile stimulation
- Range of motion
- Promote physical stretching and movement of muscles

Materials:

- 1 old sheet or tarp
- 3 rolls of duct tape - three different colors
- 5 Frisbees of the same color
- 5 Frisbees of a different color

Prerequisite Skills:

Every person has his or her own unique physical/cognitive abilities and needs. How a participant responds to an activity will dictate how the caregiver will modify or adapt a Lesson Plan to meet individual participant needs and abilities – now and in the future.

Program Name: Disc Tic Tac Toss   **Date:** _____

Leader: _____   **Time:** _____

Activity Outline:

Explain to the participant that you will be playing Tic Tac Toe

Game Preparation:
1. Lay the sheet out flat on the ground or table.
2. Use the first color of duct tape to mark a 3' x 3' grid on the tarp or sheet.
3. Use the second color of duct tape to mark an "X" on 5 Frisbees.
4. Use the third color of duct to tape to mark an "O" on the other 5 Frisbees.

Playing the Game:
1. Throw the Frisbees as markers to play a game of Tic Tac Toe.

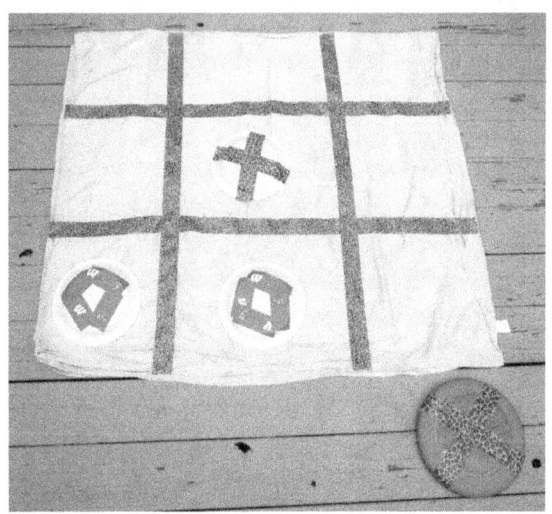

Evaluation:

Program Name: Balloon Hockey   **Date:** _____

Leader: _____   **Time:** _____

Objective:

1. Maintain/increase motor skills
2. Promote kinesthetic, sensory, visual and tactile stimulation
3. Range of motion
4. Promote physical stretching and movement of muscles

Materials:

1. Balloons
2. Long cardboard tube for each player - wrapping paper tubes work great
3. Piece of cardboard for each tube that is approximately 8" x 6"
4. Packing or duct tape
5. Large box, basket, crate or similar object that will act as the goal

Prerequisite Skills:

Every person has his or her own unique physical/cognitive abilities and needs. How a participant responds to an activity will dictate how the caregiver will modify or adapt a Lesson Plan to meet individual participant needs and abilities – now and in the future.

Program Name: Balloon Hockey   **Date:** _____

Leader: _____ **Time:** _____

Activity Outline:

Explain to the participant that you will be playing hockey.

Game Preparation:
1. To make the hockey stick, cut two slits - approximately 3 inches long down the sides of the paper tube.
2. Slide the ends of the card board into each slit.
3. Place a strip of duct tape over the area where the paper tube intersects with the cardboard piece - this will help with the sturdiness.
4. Place a strip of duct tape across the tube on both sides to secure it to the cardboard.
5. Place a couple of strips of duct tape or packing tape along the bottom of the cardboard to help with the sturdiness.
6. Inflate one balloon. The balloon will be used as the hockey puck.

Play the Game:
1. Using the cardboard hockey sticks, attempt to hit the balloon into the goal (which is the box, basket, crate or bag).

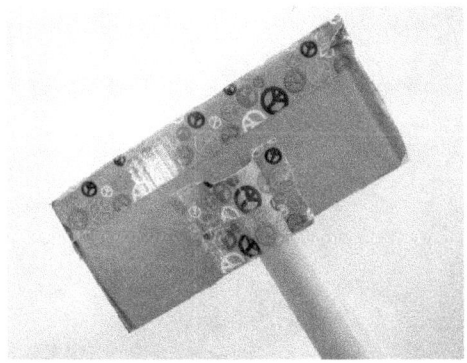 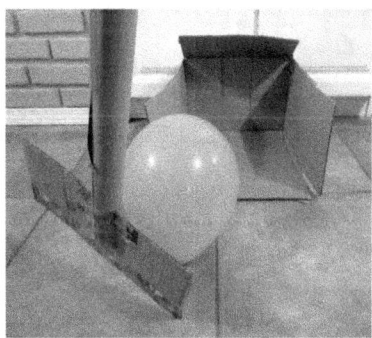

Evaluation:

Program Name: Fit Ball

Date: _____

Leader: _____

Time: _____

Objective:

- Maintain/increase motor skills
- Promote kinesthetic, sensory, visual and tactile stimulation
- Range of motion
- Promote physical stretching and movement of muscles

Materials:

- 1 large vinyl ball - see photo on pg. 67
- 1 black permanent marker

Prerequisite Skills:

Every person has his or her own unique physical/cognitive abilities and needs. How a participant responds to an activity will dictate how the caregiver will modify or adapt a Lesson Plan to meet individual participant needs and abilities – now and in the future.

Program Name: Fit Ball _____   **Date:** _____

Leader: _____   **Time:** _____

Activity Outline:

Explain to the participant that you will be playing a throwing exercise game.

1. Use the marker to write different exercises on different areas of the vinyl ball.
   - Arm Circles
   - Elbow Bends
   - Ankle Circles
   - Leg Kicks
   - Toe Taps
   - Marching
2. Hand, toss, bounce or volley the ball from one person to the next.
3. Randomly stop passing the ball. The person last holding the FitBall will pick the fitness activity that is closest to their right thumb.
4. Complete the chosen fitness activity. Continue to pass the ball back and forth, continuing to stop on occasion to do more exercise activities.

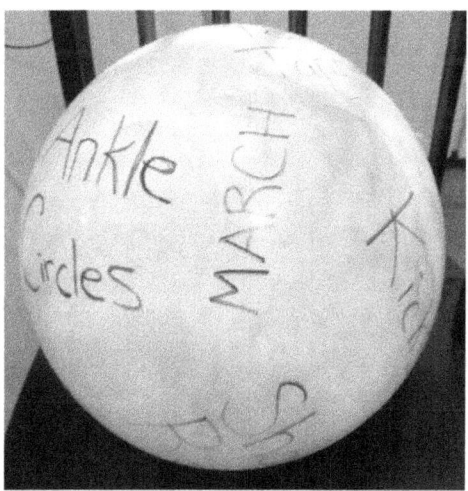

Evaluation:

Program Name: Bucket Ball   **Date:** _____

Leader: _____   **Time:** _____

Objective:

- Maintain/increase motor skills
- Promote kinesthetic, sensory, visual and tactile stimulation
- Range of motion
- Promote physical stretching and movement of muscles

Materials:

- 4 - 6 plastic buckets
- 4 - 6 nuts and bolts
- Drill
- Drill bit
- Large board - big enough for the buckets to sit on
- Black permanent market
- Paint (optional)

Prerequisite Skills:

Every person has his or her own unique physical/cognitive abilities and needs. How a participant responds to an activity will dictate how the caregiver will modify or adapt a Lesson Plan to meet individual participant needs and abilities – now and in the future.

Program Name: Bucket Ball   **Date:** _____

Leader: _____   **Time:** _____

Activity Outline:

Explain to the participant that you will be playing a throwing accuracy game.

Game Preparation:
1. Find a board big enough to sit all your buckets on. (These directions use 6 buckets, but you can do less or more).
2. Paint the board whatever color you want. (optional)
3. Place buckets on the board and trace around them.
4. Drill a hole in the center of each circle that is traced on board.
5. Stack all of the buckets together. Drill a hole through the bottom of the buckets. Stacking the buckets will prevent the buckets from splitting!
6. Unstack the buckets after the hole is drilled through them.
7. Place the bolt on the bottom of the board and then place the bucket on top of it. Thread on the nut inside the bucket. Repeat with the remaining buckets.
8. Using paint or a market, write numbers onto the buckets to represent the point value.
9. Use a ping pong ball, bouncy ball or bean bag to throw into the buckets.

Evaluation:

Activity Lesson Plans

Cooking Fun

Cooking Fun Tips

- The leader must always be present when engaged in an activity.

- The leader must take all necessary and reasonable precautions to ensure the safety of the participant.

- The leader should have necessary materials ready and prepared prior to beginning the activity.

- To ensure that the participant reaps the benefits of being engaged, please adapt any and all activities to the participant's functional level.

- The leader should read all step-by-step directions of an Activity Outline before beginning an activity with a participant. The step-by-step directions are general guidelines for the leader/caregiver to use and potentially modify in order to help the participant successfully engage in the chosen activity.

- The leader must allow for the participant to be successful. The leader may have to do all prep work, mixing and cooking depending on the participant's cognitive and physical abilities. It will be up to the leader to adjust their level of involvement so that the participant does engage in these activities.

- If mistakes are made by participant in areas such as measuring ingredients - do not criticize or intimidate the participant.

Program Name: Shirley Temple Cupcakes   **Date:** _____

Leader: _____   **Time:** _____

Objective:

- Maintain/increase motor skills
- Tactile, olfactory and visual stimulation
- Cognitive and memory stimulation
- Having fun

Materials:

- 1½ cups plus 1 tablespoon flour
- 1 teaspoon baking powder
- ½ teaspoon salt
- ½ cup unsalted butter, at room temperature
- 1 cup granulated sugar
- 2 large eggs
- ½ cup 7-Up
- 1 teaspoon pure vanilla extract
- 1 tablespoon maraschino cherry juice
- Several drops of red food coloring
- 1 12-well muffin pan
- 12 cupcake liners
- 2 mixing bowls
- Whisk
- Oven mitt
- Large print copy of recipe

Note: If mistakes are made by the participant in areas such as measuring ingredients - do not criticize the participant.

Prerequisite Skills:

Every person has his or her own unique physical/cognitive abilities and needs. How a participant responds to an activity will dictate how the caregiver will modify or adapt a Lesson Plan to meet individual participant needs and abilities – now and in the future.

Program Name: <u>Shirley Temple Cupcakes</u>   **Date**: _____

Leader: _____   **Time**: _____

Activity Outline:

Explain to the participant that together, you will be making cupcakes.

1. Provide large print copy of recipe.
2. Set out all needed materials.
3. Preheat oven to 350 degrees.
4. Line the cupcake tray with cupcake liners.
5. In a large mixing bowl, whisk together 1 ½ cups of flour, baking powder and salt.
6. In a second bowl, cream the butter and sugar together until light and fluffy.
7. Add the eggs one at a time to the butter and sugar mixture, continuing to mix after each addition.
8. Add half the flour mixture, the 7-Up and then the rest of the flour mixture - continue mixing.
9. Add the vanilla extract and continue mixing. *Do not be concerned if the batter looks a bit curdled.
10. Take a ½ cup of the batter and put in a small bowl.
11. Add the remaining 1 tablespoon of flour, the maraschino cherry juice and enough red food coloring to turn the batter red to the small bowl. Stir well.
12. Divide the red batter evenly when adding it into the cupcake liners (about 1 big teaspoon per cupcake liner).
13. Spoon the batter from the second bowl on top of the red batter, trying not to mix the two colors, but to keep in layers.
14. Bake for 15 – 20 minutes or until the tops of the cupcakes are slightly springy and a toothpick inserted into the center comes out clean.
15. Using an oven mitt, remove the pan from the oven.
16. Let cool in the pan for 5 minutes then remove to a wire rack to finish cooling before frosting. (The cupcakes will puff up a bit while cooking because of the 7-Up.)

Note: The leader may have to do all prep work, mixing and cooking depending on the participant's cognitive and physical abilities.

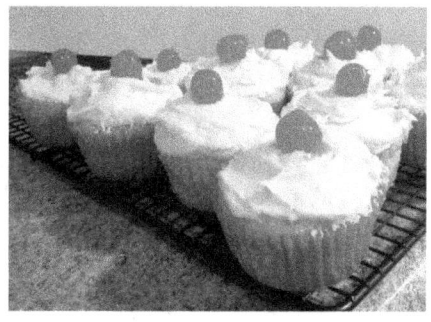

Evaluation:

Program Name: Cherry Frosting _____ **Date:** _____

Leader: _____ **Time:** _____

Objective:

- Maintain/increase motor skills
- Tactile, olfactory and visual stimulation
- Cognitive and memory stimulation
- Having fun

Materials:

- ½ cup unsalted butter, at room temperature
- 1 large pinch salt
- 2½ cups confectioner's sugar
- ½ teaspoon pure vanilla extract
- 1 teaspoon freshly squeezed juice of lemon
- 1 tablespoon maraschino cherry juice
- Mixing bowl
- Whisk
- Mixing spoon
- Large print copy of recipe

Prerequisite Skills:

Every person has his or her own unique physical/cognitive abilities and needs. How a participant responds to an activity will dictate how the caregiver will modify or adapt a Lesson Plan to meet individual participant needs and abilities – now and in the future.

Program Name: <u>Cherry Frosting</u>   **Date:** _____

Leader: _____   **Time:** _____

Activity Outline:

Explain to the participant that together, you will be making cherry frosting.

1. Provide large print copy of recipe.
2. Set out all needed materials.
3. In a mixing bowl, beat the butter and salt until creamy.
4. Sift in the confectioner's sugar and mix on low until fully combined.
5. Add the vanilla, lemon juice and maraschino cherry juice. Mix to combine.
6. Frost the cupcakes with the frosting and top each cupcake with a maraschino cherry.

Note: The leader must allow for the participant to be successful. The leader may have to do all prep work, mixing and cooking depending on the participant's cognitive and physical abilities. It will be up to leader to adjust their level of involvement so that the participant does engage in this activity.

Note: If mistakes are made by the participant in areas such as measuring ingredients - do not criticize the participant.

Evaluation:

Program Name: Pool Party Jell-O   **Date:** _____

Leader: _____   **Time:** _____

Objective:

- Maintain/increase motor skills
- Tactile, olfactory and visual stimulation
- Cognitive and memory stimulation
- Having fun

Materials:

- 6 oz. box of blue Jell-O
- 1 small container whipped topping
- 1 package of Gummy Bears
- Paper umbrellas
- Clear plastic cups
- Disposable icing bag
- Large print copy of recipe
- Spoons

Prerequisite Skills:

Every person has his or her own unique physical/cognitive abilities and needs. How a participant responds to an activity will dictate how the caregiver will modify or adapt a Lesson Plan to meet individual participant needs and abilities – now and in the future.

Program Name: Pool Party Jell-O   **Date:** _____

Leader: _____   **Time:** _____

Activity Outline:

Explain to the participant that together, you will be making a sweet treat.

1. Provide large print copy of recipe.
2. Set out all needed materials.
3. Combine Jell-O powder with 2½ cups of boiling water and stir until dissolved.
4. Pour Jell-O into individual cups and refrigerate according to directions on box.
5. An hour before serving, put the whipped topping in a disposable icing bag and snip the tip off.
6. Pipe the whipped topping onto half of the Jell-O in each cup.
7. Place the gummy bears on the whipped topping.
8. Open a paper umbrella and stick into the whipped topping.

9. Grab a spoon and enjoy!

Note: The leader must allow for participant to be successful. The leader may have to do all prep work, mixing and cooking depending on the participant's cognitive and physical abilities. It will be up to leader to adjust their level of involvement so that the participant does engage in this activity.

Note: If mistakes are made by the participant in areas such as measuring ingredients - do not criticize the participant.

Evaluation:

Program Name: Oreo & Peanut Butter Brownie Cake   **Date:** _____

Leader: _____   **Time:** _____

Objective:

- Maintain/increase motor skills
- Tactile, olfactory and visual stimulation
- Cognitive and memory stimulation
- Having fun

Materials:

- 1 box of brownie mix
- ½ cup of creamy peanut butter
- 1 package of Oreos
- 1 12-well muffin pan
- 12 cupcake liners
- 1 measuring teaspoon
- 1 measuring Tablespoon
- Large print copy of recipe

Note: The leader must allow for participant to be successful. The leader may have to do all prep work, mixing and cooking depending on the participant's cognitive and physical abilities. It will be up to the leader to adjust their level of involvement so that the participant does engage in this activity.

Note: If mistakes are made by participant in areas such as measuring ingredients - do not criticize the participant.

Prerequisite Skills:

Every person has his or her own unique physical/cognitive abilities and needs. How a participant responds to an activity will dictate how the caregiver will modify or adapt a Lesson Plan to meet individual participant needs and abilities – now and in the future.

Program Name: Oreo & Peanut Butter Brownie Cake   **Date:** _____

Leader: _____   **Time:** _____

Activity Outline:

Explain to the participant that together, you will be making a sweet treat.

1. Provide large print copy of recipe.
2. Set out all needed materials.
3. Preheat the oven to 350 degrees.
4. Prepare the brownie mix according to the package instructions.
5. Take 24 Oreos out from their package.
6. Put 1 teaspoon of peanut butter over the first Oreo.
7. Press a second Oreo on top of the first.
8. Put one teaspoon of peanut butter on top of the second Oreo.
9. Place the stack of Oreos into a cupcake liner in the muffin pan.
10. Continue steps 2 through 5 for the remaining Oreos.
11. Take the brownie mix and pour 2 tablespoons of the mix onto the top of the Oreo stack, letting the mix run down the sides of the cookies.
12. Bake for 18-20 minutes.
13. Cool completely before serving.

Evaluation:

Program Name: American Pie-in-a-Jar   **Date:** _____

Leader: _____   **Time:** _____

Objective:

- Maintain/increase motor skills
- Tactile, olfactory and visual stimulation
- Range of motion
- Cognitive and memory stimulation

Materials:

- 8 – 10 oz. glass canning jars
- 1 can of blueberry OR cherry pie filling
- 1 package of pie dough
- Small star-shaped cookie cutter
- 1/3 cup of sugar
- 1 fork
- 1 spoon or 1 tablespoon
- 1/2 teaspoon
- 1 rimmed baking sheet
- Oven mitt
- Large print copy of recipe

Note: The leader must allow for the participant to be successful. The leader may have to do all prep work, mixing and cooking depending on the participant's cognitive and physical abilities. It will be up to the leader to adjust their level of involvement so that the participant does engage in this activity.

Note: If mistakes are made by the participant in areas such as measuring ingredients - do not criticize the participant.

Prerequisite Skills:

Every person has his or her own unique physical/cognitive abilities and needs. How a participant responds to an activity will dictate how the caregiver will modify or adapt a Lesson Plan to meet individual participant needs and abilities – now and in the future.

Program Name: American Pie-in-a-Jar_____   **Date:** _____

Leader: _____   **Time:** _____

Activity Outline:

Explain to the participant that together, you will be making a sweet treat.

1. Provide a large print copy of recipe.
2. Set out all needed materials.
3. Preheat oven to 400 degrees.
4. Place a rimmed baking sheet into the oven to preheat.
5. Liberally butter the canning jars.
6. For the bottom crusts, cut out a 5" square from the pie dough and press into the bottom of the jar.
7. For the tops, use a canning jar to press out a circle.
8. Use the scraps to cut out the stars with a small cookie cutter.
9. Spoon in 4 tablespoons or so of the pie filling and press the top crust into place, crimping the edges with a fork.
10. Add the star to the top and make four very small incisions in the top of the dough to vent.
11. Sprinkle the top of each pie with ½ teaspoon of sugar.
12. Place the prepared pies onto the heated cookie sheet and bake for 20 minutes.
13. Using an oven mitt, turn the cookie sheet, decrease oven temperature to 350 degrees, and bake for another 10 minutes until the crust is golden brown and the filling is bubbling.
14. Remove from the oven using an oven mitt. Allow to cool completely before serving.

Evaluation:

Program Name: Mississippi Mud Puddles   **Date:** _____

Leader: _____   **Time:** _____

Objective:

- Maintain/increase motor skills
- Tactile, olfactory and visual stimulation
- Cognitive and memory stimulation
- Having fun

Materials:

- 1 cup flour
- 1 stick butter
- 1 cup chopped pecans
- 1 package semi-sweet chocolate chips
- 8 ounce cream cheese
- 1 pint heavy cream
- 1 cup powdered sugar
- 1 cup whipped topping
- 1 large box of instant chocolate pudding mix
- 1 large box of instant French vanilla pudding mix
- 5 cups milk
- 6 ounce clear, plastic cups
- 1 9x13" pan
- 3 mixing bowls
- Mixing spoon
- Large print copy of recipe
- Oven mitt

Note: If mistakes are made by participant in areas such as measuring ingredients - do not criticize the participant.

Note: Leader may have to do all prep work and mixing depending on the participant's cognitive and physical abilities.

Prerequisite Skills:

Every person has his or her own unique physical/cognitive abilities and needs. How a participant responds to an activity will dictate how the caregiver will modify or adapt a Lesson Plan to meet individual participant needs and abilities – now and in the future.

Program Name: Mississippi Mud Puddles   **Date:** _____

Leader: _____   **Time:** _____

Activity Outline:

Explain to the participant that together, you will be making a sweet treat.

1. Provide large print copy of recipe.
2. Set out all needed materials.
3. Preheat the oven to 375 degrees.
4. Prepare the components first and then begin assembly- the layers will be:
   - A. Crust
   - B. White Cream Cheese Fluff
   - C. Chocolate Pudding
   - D. French Vanilla Pudding
   - E. Ganache
   - F. Whipped topping
3. Mix 2 ½ cups of milk with the French vanilla pudding mix and refrigerate.
4. Mix 2 ½ cups of milk with the chocolate pudding mix and refrigerate.
5. Crust - Combine one cup of flour, one stick of melted butter and one cup of chopped pecans. Press into a 9x13 pan. Bake for 15 minutes.
6. Using oven mitts, remove pan from the oven and let cool.
7. Cream Cheese Fluff - Combine cream cheese, powdered sugar and the whipped topping. Hand mix until smooth.
8. Ganache - Melt the chocolate chips and heavy cream together - this can be done in the microwave. Stir together until silky smooth.
9. Begin assembly - Spoon some of the crust into the plastic dessert cups - just crumble it up.
10. Add one layer of the cream cheese fluff.
11. Next, add one layer of the chocolate pudding.
12. Now add one layer of the French vanilla pudding.
13. Add one layer of the ganache (make sure the ganache is cool before adding to the layers)
14. Top with whipped topping and a few chocolate chips.

Evaluation:

Program Name: Grasshopper Parfaits   **Date:** _____

Leader: _____   **Time:** _____

Objective:

- Maintain/increase motor skills
- Tactile, olfactory and visual stimulation
- Cognitive and memory stimulation
- Having fun

Materials:

- 15 Oreo cookies
- 10 chocolate covered mint patties
- 2 - 3.9 ounce packages of instant chocolate pudding mix
- 4 cups cold milk
- 12 drops green food coloring
- 2 cups whipped topping
- 2 1-gallon Ziploc bags
- 2 large mixing bowls
- Whisk
- Large print copy of recipe
- 12 clear plastic cups

Prerequisite Skills:

Every person has his or her own unique physical/cognitive abilities and needs. How a participant responds to an activity will dictate how the caregiver will modify or adapt a Lesson Plan to meet individual participant needs and abilities – now and in the future.

Program Name: Grasshopper Parfaits   **Date:** _____

Leader: _____   **Time:** _____

Activity Outline:

Explain to the participant that you will be making a sweet treat

1. Provide large print copy of recipe.
2. Set out all needed materials.
3. Place the 15 Oreo cookies into a 1-Gallon Ziploc Bag and break/crush into small pieces.
4. Place the 10 chocolate covered mint patties into the other 1-Gallon Ziploc Bag and break/crush into small pieces.
5. Combine Oreo cookie pieces and mint patty pieces in a mixing bowl.
6. Beat pudding mixes and milk with a whisk for 2 minutes. Let stand for 5 minutes.
7. Stir 12 drops of green food coloring into the 2 cups of whipped topping.
8. Put one layer of the chocolate pudding at the bottom of the clear, plastic glass.
9. Add one layer of the whipped topping.
10. Place a thin layer of the crushed cookies.
11. Repeat a layer of the chocolate pudding, then the whipped topping and top with a thin layer of crushed cookies.
12. Repeat steps 8 - 10 in eleven more plastic cups.

Note: The leader must allow for the participant to be successful. The leader may have to do all prep work, mixing, and cooking depending on the participant's cognitive and physical abilities. It will be up to the leader to adjust their level of involvement so that the participant does engage in this activity.

Note: If mistakes are made by the participant in areas such as measuring ingredients - do not criticize the participant.

Evaluation:

Program Name: Banana Split Bites   **Date:** _____

Leader: _____   **Time:** _____

Objective:

- Maintain/increase motor skills
- Tactile, olfactory and visual stimulation
- Cognitive and memory stimulation
- Having fun

Materials:

- 3 bananas
- 1/4 lb. cored pineapple
- 6 strawberries
- 1 cup dipping chocolate
- 1/4 cup chopped peanuts (optional)
- 12 popsicle sticks (or skewers)
- Large print copy of recipe
- Microwave safe bowl
- 9x13 baking sheet
- Paring knife
- Wax paper or parchment paper
- Plate (if using chopped peanuts)

Note: The leader must allow for the participant to be successful. The leader may have to do all prep work, mixing, and cooking depending on the participant's cognitive and physical abilities. It will be up to the leader to adjust their level of involvement so that the participant does engage in this activity.

Note: If mistakes are made by the participant in areas such as measuring ingredients - do not criticize the participant.

Prerequisite Skills:

Every person has his or her own unique physical/cognitive abilities and needs. How a participant responds to an activity will dictate how the caregiver will modify or adapt a Lesson Plan to meet individual participant needs and abilities – now and in the future.

Program Name: Banana Split Bites _____ **Date:** _____

Leader: _____ **Time:** _____

Activity Outline:

Explain to the participant that together, you will be making a sweet treat.

1. Provide large print copy of recipe.
2. Set out all needed materials.
3. Cut strawberries in half.
4. For each strawberry half, cut an equal size piece of banana and pineapple.
5. Place pineapple on the skewer first, then the banana and lastly the strawberry.
6. Place in freezer for 10 minutes.
7. Line a tray with wax paper or parchment paper.
8. Put chopped nuts in small plate to use for dipping. (optional)
9. Melt chocolate by heating in microwave for 30 seconds, stirring and repeating until melted and smooth.
10. Dip cold fruit in chocolate, then into nuts, then place on prepared tray.

Evaluation:

Program Name: Cheesecake Stuffed Strawberry Bites   **Date:** _____

Leader: _____   **Time:** _____

Objective:

- Maintain/increase motor skills
- Tactile, olfactory and visual stimulation
- Cognitive and memory stimulation
- Having fun

Materials:

- 1 lb. large strawberries
- 8 ounces cream cheese, softened
- 3-4 tablespoons powdered sugar
- 1 teaspoon vanilla extract
- Graham cracker crumbs
- Large print copy of recipe
- Paring knife
- Mixing bowl
- Disposable pastry bag or Zip-loc bag
- Hand mixer or stand mixer

Note: The leader must allow for the participant to be successful. The leader may have to do all prep work, mixing and cooking depending on the participant's cognitive and physical abilities. It will be up to the leader to adjust their level of involvement so that the participant does engage in this activity.

Note: If mistakes are made by the participant in areas such as measuring ingredients - do not criticize the participant.

Prerequisite Skills:

Every person has his or her own unique physical/cognitive abilities and needs. How a participant responds to an activity will dictate how the caregiver will modify or adapt a Lesson Plan to meet individual participant needs and abilities – now and in the future.

Program Name: Cheesecake Stuffed Strawberry Bites   **Date:** _____

Leader: _____   **Time:** _____

Activity Outline:

Explain to the participant that together, you will be making a sweet treat.

1. Provide large print copy of recipe.
2. Set out all needed materials.
3. Rinse strawberries.
4. Cut around the top of the strawberry and remove the top.
5. Clean out with a paring knife, if necessary (some may already be hollow inside).
6. Set aside the strawberries.
7. In a mixing bowl, beat the cream cheese, powdered sugar and vanilla until creamy.
8. Add the cream cheese mix to a piping bag. (If you don't have a piping bag, simply use a Ziploc bag with the corner cut off.)
9. Fill the strawberries with the cheesecake mixture.
10. Once strawberries are filled, dip the top in graham cracker crumbs.
11. If not serving immediately, refrigerate until serving.

Evaluation:

Program Name: Patriotic Ice Cream Cones   **Date:** _____

Leader: _____   **Time:** _____

Objective:

- Maintain/increase motor skills
- Tactile and visual stimulation
- Cognitive and memory stimulation
- Having fun

Materials:

- Sugar ice cream cones
- 2 cups of white chocolate chips or milk chocolate chips
- 1/2 cup of butter
- Red, white and blue sprinkles
- Small saucepan
- Wooden spoon
- 3 small bowls
- 1 larger bowl
- Wax paper
- Pastry brush (optional)
- Large print copy of recipe

Note: The leader must allow for the participant to be successful. The leader may have to do all prep work, mixing and cooking depending on the participant's cognitive and physical abilities. It will be up to the leader to adjust their level of involvement so that the participant does engage in this activity.

Note: If mistakes are made by the participant in areas such as measuring ingredients - do not criticize the participant.

Prerequisite Skills:

Every person has his or her own unique physical/cognitive abilities and needs. How a participant responds to an activity will dictate how the caregiver will modify or adapt a Lesson Plan to meet individual participant needs and abilities – now and in the future.

Program Name: Patriotic Ice Cream Cones   **Date:** _____

Leader: _____   **Time:** _____

Activity Outline:

Explain to the participant that together, you will be turning good ice cream cones into GREAT ice cream cones.

1. Provide large print copy of recipe.
2. Set out all needed materials.
3. Melt butter and chocolate chips of your choice in small saucepan over low heat, stirring constantly.
4. When chocolate is completely melted, transfer to larger bowl immediately.
5. Either dip top of ice cream cone into melted chocolate or paint the chocolate on the cones using a pastry brush.
6. Immediately sprinkle on the décor.
7. Set the cones on wax paper to dry and cool.

Evaluation:

Program Name: Jell-O Firecrackers   **Date:** _____

Leader: _____   **Time:** _____

Objective:

- Maintain/increase motor skills
- Tactile and visual stimulation
- Cognitive and memory stimulation
- Having fun

Materials:

- 1 - 3 ounce package blue Jell-O
- 1 - 3 ounce package red Jell-O
- 1 envelope of unflavored Gelatin
- 1 cup of milk
- 3 tablespoons sugar
- ½ teaspoon vanilla
- 20 maraschino cherries
- 1 1/3 cups water
- 20 plastic shot glasses
- Cooking spray
- 3 small bowls
- 1 saucepan
- Large print copy of recipe

Prerequisite Skills:

Every person has his or her own unique physical/cognitive abilities and needs. How a participant responds to an activity will dictate how the caregiver will modify or adapt a Lesson Plan to meet individual participant needs and abilities – now and in the future.

Program Name: Jell-O Firecrackers _____ **Date**: _____

Leader: _____ **Time**: _____

Activity Outline:

Explain to the participant that you will be making a fabulous sweet treat.

1. Provide large print copy of recipe.
2. Set out all needed materials.
3. Add 2/3 cup boiling water to the blue Jell-O mix and stir until completely dissolved.
4. Repeat Step 1 in a separate bowl with the red Jell-O mix.
5. In a separate bowl, add the unflavored gelatin and ¼ cup milk - let stand for 5 minutes.
6. Add the remaining milk to a saucepan and bring to a simmer.
7. Remove the saucepan from heat and add the vanilla and sugar
8. Add this to the plain gelatin mixture and stir until the gelatin is completely dissolved.
9. Lightly spray the plastic shot glasses with cooking spray.
10. Spoon about 2 teaspoons of the blue Jell-O into each glass and refrigerate for 15 minutes.
11. Top with about 2 teaspoons of the unflavored gelatin mix and refrigerate for 10 minutes.
12. Place a cherry, stem up, into the white gelatin layer in each cup and refrigerate for 2 minutes.
13. Cover with about 2 teaspoons of the red Jell-O and refrigerate for 2 hours.
14. Remove the desserts from the cups before serving.

Note: The leader must allow for the participant to be successful. The leader may have to do all prep work, mixing, and cooking depending on the participant's cognitive and physical abilities. It will be up to the leader to adjust their level of involvement so that the participant does engage in this activity.

Note: If mistakes are made by the participant in areas such as measuring ingredients - do not criticize the participant.

Evaluation:

Program Name: Berry Hand Pies   **Date:** _____

Leader: _____   **Time:** _____

Objective:

- Maintain/increase motor skills
- Tactile and visual stimulation
- Cognitive and memory stimulation
- Having fun

Materials:

- Ready made pie dough (unroll, fill and bake)
- Pie filling - any berry flavor
- All-purpose flour for dusting
- 1 egg
- Small bowl
- Whisk
- Star shaped cookie cutter
- Parchment paper
- Baking sheet
- Fork
- Pastry brush
- Large print copy of recipe
- Oven mitt

Prerequisite Skills:

Every person has his or her own unique physical/cognitive abilities and needs. How a participant responds to an activity will dictate how the caregiver will modify or adapt a Lesson Plan to meet individual participant needs and abilities – now and in the future.

Program Name: Berry Hand Pies   **Date:** _____

Leader: _____   **Time:** _____

Activity Outline:

Explain to the participant that you will be making a fabulous sweet treat.

1. Provide large print copy of recipe.
2. Set out all needed materials.
3. Preheat the oven to 375 degrees.
4. On a lightly floured surface, roll out the ready-made pie dough.
5. Use a cookie cutter to cut-out star shapes from the pie dough.
6. Repeat the process until all of the dough has been used. You will need an even number of stars as half will be the pie tops and half will be the bottoms.
7. Place the stars on a parchment lined baking sheet.
8. Place a scoop of pie filling in the center of each pie bottom.
9. Cover the pie bottoms with the stars you have saved for the pie tops and seal by pressing the edges together with a fork.
10. Whisk the egg in a small bowl. Using a pastry brush, brush the sealed pies with the egg.
11. Bake the pies for about 25 minutes - until the berry filling bubbles and the crust is browned.
12. Using an oven mitt, remove pies from the oven and set aside to cool.
13. Serve and enjoy!

Note: The leader must allow for the participant to be successful. The leader may have to do all prep work, mixing, and cooking depending on the participant's cognitive and physical abilities. It will be up to the leader to adjust their level of involvement so that the participant does engage in this activity.

Note: If mistakes are made by the participant in areas such as measuring ingredients - do not criticize the participant.

Evaluation:

Program Name: Zucchini Boats _____ **Date:** _____

Leader: _____ **Time:** _____

Objective:

- Maintain/increase motor skills
- Tactile, olfactory and visual stimulation
- Range of motion
- Cognitive and memory stimulation
- Having fun

Materials:
- 1 zucchini
- Olive oil
- Salt
- Pepper
- 1 small package of grape tomatoes
- Bread crumbs
- 1 package of mozzarella cheese - cubed
- Grated parmesan
- Knife
- Baking dish
- Spoon
- Large print copy of recipe
- Pastry brush
- Oven mitt

Note: The leader must allow for the participant to be successful. The leader may have to do all prep work, mixing, and cooking depending on the participant's cognitive and physical abilities. It will be up to the leader to adjust their level of involvement so that the participant does engage in these activity.

Note: If mistakes are made by participant in areas such as measuring ingredients - do not criticize the participant.

Prerequisite Skills:

Every person has his or her own unique physical/cognitive abilities and needs. How a participant responds to an activity will dictate how the caregiver will modify or adapt a Lesson Plan to meet individual participant needs and abilities – now and in the future.

Program Name: Zucchini Boats   **Date:** _____

Leader: _____   **Time:** _____

Activity Outline:

Explain to the participant that you will be making a snack.

1. Preheat the oven to 350 degrees.
2. Cut zucchini in half-length wise and then trim a bit off of the bottom so it will lay flat in the baking dish. Place zucchini in the baking dish.
3. Use the spoon to scoop out the seeds from the center of the zucchini.
4. Using a pastry brush, brush the top of the zucchini with a mixture of olive oil, salt and pepper.
5. Cut the grape tomatoes in half and place them on top of the zucchini, in between the grooves.
6. Sprinkle bread crumbs over the top of the zucchini.
7. Place in oven and cook for 30 minutes.
8. Remove the baking dish from the oven and place the cubed mozzarella cheese between the grape tomatoes on the zucchini.
9. Place baking dish back in oven and switch the oven to broil.
10. Watch for the top of the zucchini to turn golden and for the cheese to bubble - about 5 minutes - this time will vary by oven.
11. Using an oven mitt, remove the baking dish from the oven and drizzle with olive oil and a sprinkle of grated parmesan cheese.

Evaluation:

Program Name: Individual Seven Layer Dips   **Date:** _____

Leader: _____   **Time:** _____

Objective:

- Maintain/increase motor skills
- Tactile, olfactory and visual stimulation
- Range of motion
- Cognitive and memory stimulation
- Having fun

Materials:

- 16 ounce can refried beans
- 1 ounce package taco seasoning
- 1 cup guacamole
- 8 ounces sour cream
- 1 cup chunky salsa
- 1 cup shredded cheddar cheese
- 2 Roma tomatoes, diced
- ½ bunch green onions, sliced
- 2.25 ounce can of sliced black olives, drained
- 8 - nine ounce plastic tumblers
- Tortilla chips

Prerequisite Skills:

Every person has his or her own unique physical/cognitive abilities and needs. How a participant responds to an activity will dictate how the caregiver will modify or adapt a Lesson Plan to meet individual participant needs and abilities – now and in the future.

Program Name: Individual Seven Layer Dips   **Date:** _____

Leader: _____   **Time:** _____

Activity Outline:

Explain to the participant that you will be making a snack dip

1. In a small bowl, mix the taco seasoning and refried beans.
2. In each plastic glass, layer about 2 tablespoons of the beans.
3. Layer 2 tablespoons of sour cream.
4. Next, layer 2 tablespoons of guacamole.
5. Now, layer 2 tablespoons of salsa or Pico de Gallo. Be sure to drain the salsa or Pico de Gallo to remove the excess liquid before layering.
6. Next, layer 2 tablespoons of cheese.
7. Finally, top with 1-2 teaspoons of tomatoes, olives, and green onion. (If making ahead of time, wait to add these toppings until shortly before serving.)
8. Store in the refrigerator until serving. Serve with chips. Makes around 8 individual dips.

Note: The leader must allow for the participant to be successful. The leader may have to do all prep work, mixing, and cooking depending on the participant's cognitive and physical abilities. It will be up to the leader to adjust their level of involvement so that the participant does engage in this activity.

Note: If mistakes are made by the participant in areas such as measuring ingredients - do not criticize the participant.

Evaluation:

Activity Lesson Plans

Patriotic Projects

God Bless America Crafts and Stuff Tips

- The leader must always be present when engaged in an activity.

- The leader must take all necessary and reasonable precautions to ensure the safety of the participant.

- The leader should have necessary materials ready and prepared prior to beginning the activity.

- To ensure that the participant reaps the benefits of being engaged, please adapt any and all activities to the participant's functional level.

- The leader should read all step-by-step directions of an Activity Outline before beginning an activity with a participant. The step-by-step directions are general guidelines for the leader/caregiver to use and potentially modify in order to help the participant successfully engage in the chosen activity.

- The leader must allow for participant to be successful. The leader may have to do all of the prep work depending on the participant's cognitive and physical abilities. It will be up to the leader to adjust their level of involvement so that the participant does engage in these activities.

- If mistakes are made by the participant - do not criticize the participant.

Program Name: Patriotic Rag Wreath _____ **Date:** _____

Leader: _____ **Time:** _____

Objective:

- Maintain/increase motor skills
- Tactile and visual stimulation
- Reminisce
- Having fun

Materials:

- 3 strips of red color fabric 7" x 48" long
- 3 strips of white color fabric 7" x 48" long
- 3 strips of blue color fabric 7" x 48" long
- Rotary cutter or scissors
- Wire wreath form
- Hot-glue gun
- Glue sticks
- Optional - embellishments (stickers)

Prerequisite Skills:

Every person has his or her own unique physical/cognitive abilities and needs. How a participant responds to an activity will dictate how the caregiver will modify or adapt a Lesson Plan to meet individual participant needs and abilities – now and in the future.

Program Name: Patriotic Rag Wreath   **Date:** _____

Leader: _____   **Time:** _____

Activity Outline:

Explain to the participant that you will be making a patriotic wreath.

1. Use the rotary cutter or scissors to cut the fabric into 1" x 7" strips.
2. Knot the fabric strips around the wire frame. Alternate red, white and blue fabrics.
3. Use a hot-glue gun to add any embellishments to the wreath.
4. Hang and admire!

Note: The closer together you push the knots - the fuller the wreath will look!

Evaluation:

Program Name: Flag Blocks   **Date:** _____

Leader: _____   **Time:** _____

Objective:

- Maintain/increase motor skills
- Tactile and visual stimulation
- Reminisce
- Having fun

Materials:

- 2 x 4 lumber cut into: 2 - 7" blocks and 4 - 3.5" blocks
- Red, white and blue craft paint
- Sandpaper
- Wood stain
- White cardstock
- 3" star stencil
- Pencil
- Distress ink
- Double-sided tape or Mod Podge
- Gold wire ribbon

Prerequisite Skills:

Every person has his or her own unique physical/cognitive abilities and needs. How a participant responds to an activity will dictate how the caregiver will modify or adapt a Lesson Plan to meet individual participant needs and abilities – now and in the future.

Program Name: Flag Blocks   **Date:** _____

Leader: _____   **Time:** _____

Activity Outline:

Explain to the participant that you will be making Patriotic Blocks.

1. Decide the configuration so you know which sides of the blocks you want to paint.
2. Paint the front, "skinny" sides of the wood; one long cream, one long red, one short cream and one short red.
3. Leave one of the remaining 3.5" blocks bare of paint and paint the bigger side of the other block blue.
4. Once the paint has dried, sand it well with sandpaper - particularly around the edges. This will fade the paint and give the blocks a weathered appearance.
5. Wipe off the dust from sanding and apply the stain.
6. Stencil the star onto the white cardstock. Distress the star with the distress ink and then cut the star shape out.
7. Adhere the star to the front of the blue block with either double sided tape or Mod Podge.
8. Stack up your blocks in the configuration you used in Step 1.
9. Tie the gold ribbon around the blocks and you are finished!

Evaluation:

Program Name: Patriotic Luminaries   **Date:** _____

Leader: _____   **Time:** _____

Objective:

- Maintain/increase motor skills
- Tactile and visual stimulation
- Reminisce
- Having fun

Materials:

- Glass jars
- Red, white and blue pleated or ruffled trim
- Twine
- Ribbon
- Scissors
- Mod Podge
- Brush
- Hot-glue gun
- Hot-glue gun glue sticks
- Tealight candle

Prerequisite Skills:

Every person has his or her own unique physical/cognitive abilities and needs. How a participant responds to an activity will dictate how the caregiver will modify or adapt a Lesson Plan to meet individual participant needs and abilities – now and in the future.

Program Name: Patriotic Luminaries   **Date:** _____

Leader: _____   **Time:** _____

Activity Outline:

Explain to the participant that you will be making Patriotic Luminaries.

1. Lay all material out so it is easily accessible.
2. Cut the ribbon and trim to fit the size of the jar.
3. Secure the end of twine with the hot-glue gun.
4. Then use the Mod Podge to glue twine to the areas of jar you want decorated. It is important to use the Mod Podge - NOT the glue gun - to adhere the twine! Mod Podge will not melt when the glass heats up from the candle.
5. Using the Mod Podge, attach the ribbon and trim in various combinations.
6. Place a candle in the luminary and enjoy the beautiful glow!

Evaluation:

Program Name: Patriotic Doily Banner   **Date:** _____

Leader: _____   **Time:** _____

Objective:

- Maintain/increase motor skills
- Tactile and visual stimulation
- Reminisce
- Having fun

Materials:

- Multiple white doilies (4", 6" & 8")
- One can of royal blue paint
- One can of red paint
- Mod Podge
- Paint brush
- Scissors
- String, ribbon or yarn to string the banner

Prerequisite Skills:

Every person has his or her own unique physical/cognitive abilities and needs. How a participant responds to an activity will dictate how the caregiver will modify or adapt a Lesson Plan to meet individual participant needs and abilities – now and in the future.

Program Name: Patriotic Doily Banner   **Date**: _____

Leader: _____   **Time**: _____

Activity Outline:

Explain to the participant that you will be making patriotic banners.

1. Lay all materials on table so they are accessible.
2. Paint the 8" doilies red.
3. Paint the 4" doilies blue.
4. After the doilies have dried, cut them in half.
5. Mod Podge the 3 layers together - the white onto the red and the blue onto the white.
6. After the Mod Podge is dry, string your yarn through the holes in the doilies.
7. Hang for decoration.

Evaluation:

Program Name: Pool Noodle Firecrackers   **Date:** _____

Leader: _____   **Time:** _____

Objective:

- Maintain/increase motor skills
- Tactile and visual stimulation
- Reminisce
- Having fun

Materials:

- Pool noodle
- Scrapbook paper
- 4th of July spray picks
- Decorative ribbon
- Mod Podge
- Foam brush
- Poly acrylic spray
- Serrated knife
- Pencil

Prerequisite Skills:

Every person has his or her own unique physical/cognitive abilities and needs. How a participant responds to an activity will dictate how the caregiver will modify or adapt a Lesson Plan to meet individual participant needs and abilities – now and in the future.

Program Name: Pool Noodle Firecrackers   **Date:** _____

Leader: _____   **Time:** _____

Activity Outline:

Explain to the participant that you will be making patriotic decorations.

1. Cut the pool noodle in half with a serrated knife.
2. Measure the scrapbook paper to fit around the pool noodle pieces.
3. Roll the paper until it wraps back around itself and draw a straight line, leaving a little to slightly overlap.
4. Spread Mod Podge on the noodle and carefully roll the paper onto the noodle. Allow to dry.
5. Cut a circle out of the paper to fit the top of the noodle. Lay the circle on the top of the noodle and poke a hole through the top with a pencil before gluing down.
6. Trim the noodle with decorative ribbon.
7. Spray with two coats of poly acrylic spray. This will give it a water resistant finish.
8. Insert the spray picks into the top and through the hole in the noodle.
9. Set out on a table for display.

Evaluation:

Program Name: Patriotic Yarn String Lights   **Date:** _____

Leader: _____   **Time:** _____

Objective:

- Maintain/increase motor skills
- Tactile and visual stimulation
- Reminisce
- Having fun

Materials:

- Red, white and blue yarn
- 1 bag of 5" balloons
- Glue
- Petroleum jelly
- 1 set of string lights
- Water
- Wire
- Shallow pan
- 2 chairs
- String
- Clothespins
- Newspaper

Prerequisite Skills:

Every person has his or her own unique physical/cognitive abilities and needs. How a participant responds to an activity will dictate how the caregiver will modify or adapt a Lesson Plan to meet individual participant needs and abilities – now and in the future.

Program Name: Patriotic Yarn String Lights _____   **Date**: _____

Leader: _____   **Time**: _____

Activity Outline:

Explain to the participant that you will be making patriotic displays.

1. Lay all materials out on table.
2. Inflate several balloons so that they are around 4" in diameter.
3. Rub petroleum jelly on the entire surface of the inflated balloons.
4. Mix 2 parts glue to 1 part water in a shallow pan. Stir until the glue mixture is smooth and even.
5. Wrap the yarn around your fingers several times. Use a small amount of yarn as you go, it is less likely to become tangled.
6. Soak the yarn in the glue mixture - keeping the yarn in a loop so it does not tangle.
7. Tie one end of the yarn loosely around the knot at the top of the balloon and start winding the yarn around the balloon.
8. Be sure to crisscross cross the yarn in different directions. When you reach the end of your yarn loop, tuck the end under another piece of yarn.
9. Now rub the entire surface with more of the glue mixture.
10. *You can use more than one color yarn at a time if you want to make each globe red, white and blue - just be sure to use the same amount of yarn for each globe.
11. Tie a piece of string between two chairs to create a drying line for the globes. Use clothespins to hang the ends of the balloons from the line. Make sure you have a row of newspaper underneath to catch the drips.
12. Allow to dry for 48 hours.
13. Pop the balloons and remove them from the yarn globes.
14. Find an opening in the globes that is large enough to insert the bulbs from your string of lights.
15. Use a small piece of wire to secure the globes to the light string. This will help them stay in place.
16. Hang and enjoy!

Evaluation:

Program Name: Red, White and Blue Mason Jars   **Date:** _____

Leader: _____   **Time:** _____

Objective:

- Maintain/increase motor skills
- Tactile and visual stimulation
- Reminisce
- Having fun

Materials:

- 3 mason jars
- One small can of Red paint
- One small can of White paint
- One small can of Blue paint
- Multiple Paint brushes
- 1 roll of Washi tape
- 4 small foam stars
- Wine cork
- Sandpaper
- Optional: Clear enamel spray

Prerequisite Skills:

Every person has his or her own unique physical/cognitive abilities and needs. How a participant responds to an activity will dictate how the caregiver will modify or adapt a Lesson Plan to meet individual participant needs and abilities – now and in the future.

Program Name: Red, White and Blue Mason Jars   **Date:** _____

Leader: _____   **Time:** _____

Activity Outline:

Explain to the participant that you will be making patriotic displays.

1. Place all materials on table so they are accessible
2. One at a time, paint mason jars
    - Paint two jars white
    - Paint one jar blue
3. Allow paint to dry.
4. Use the Washi tape to tape stripes on the two white mason jars. Try to make the tape lines as symmetrical as possible.
5. Paint the two taped jars red and set aside to dry.
    NOTE: The Washi tape will protect the white paint that is already on the jars.
6. Make a star stamp by gluing the four foam stars together and then gluing the stars on top of the wine cork. Let dry.
7. Once star stamp is dry, dip star stamp into white paint and then apply to different areas all around the mason jar that is painted blue. Let dry.
8. Remove the Washi tape from the two red jars.
9. When paint is dry on all three mason jars, distress the 3 mason jars by lightly rubbing the outside, painted surface with sandpaper.
10. Clean off jars and enjoy your patriotic displays

1. Optional - Seal the paint by spraying with a clear enamel spray.

Evaluation:

Thank you for using this edition of Caregiver Activity Lesson Plans

R.O.S. Therapy Systems offers several *Caregiver Activity Lesson Plan* books through unique partnerships with individual contributors and organizations as well as the input from the authors and staff members of R.O.S. We have amassed over hundreds of Activity Lesson Plans so that there is something for everyone:

- Craft Activities
- Holiday Activities
- Activities for Men
- Music Activities

- Gardening Activities
- Games
- Baking Activities
- Verbal Communication Skills Activities

- Outdoor Activities
- Science Activities
- Art Activities
- Computer Activities

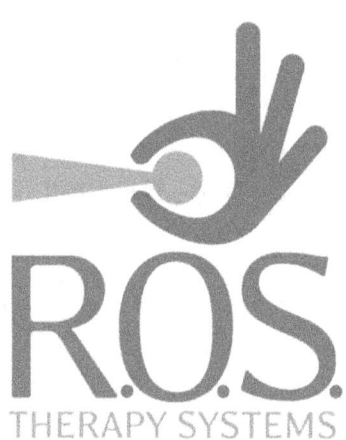